Tuberculosis Pearls

NEIL W. SCHLUGER, M.D.
Assistant Professor of Medicine
New York University School of Medicine
Director, Bellevue Hospital Chest Clinic
New York, New York

TIMOTHY J. HARKIN, M.D.
Assistant Professor of Medicine
New York University School of Medicine
Assistant Director, Bellevue Hospital Chest Service
New York, New York

Series Editors

STEVEN A. SAHN, M.D.
Professor of Medicine and Director
Division of Pulmonary and
  Critical Care Medicine
Medical University of South Carolina
Charleston, South Carolina

JOHN E. HEFFNER, M.D.
Professor of Clinical Medicine
University of Arizona Health Sciences Center
Chairman, Academic Internal Medicine
St. Joseph's Hospital and Medical Center
Phoenix, Arizona

HANLEY & BELFUS, INC./Philadelphia
MOSBY/St. Louis • Baltimore • Boston • Carlsbad • Chicago • London • Madrid
Naples • New York • Philadelphia • Sydney • Tokyo • Toronto

Publisher: HANLEY & BELFUS, INC.
                 Medical Publishers
                 210 S. 13th Street
                 Philadelphia, PA 19107
                 (215) 546-7293
                 FAX (215) 790-9330

North American and worldwide sales and distribution:

                 MOSBY
                 11830 Westline Industrial Drive
                 St. Louis, MO 63146

In Canada: Times Mirror Professional Publishing, Ltd.
                 130 Flaska Drive
                 Markham, Ontario L6G 1B8
                 Canada

Library of Congress Cataloging-in-Publication Data

Schluger, Neil W., 1959–
     Tuberculosis pearls / Neil W. Schluger, Timothy J. Harkin.
         p.   cm. — (The Pearls Series)
     Includes bibliographical references and index.
     ISBN 1-56053-156-8 (alk. paper)
     1. Tuberculosis—Case studies.   I. Harkin, Timothy J., 1959–
II. Title.   III. Series.
     [DNLM: 1. Tuberculosis, Pulmonary—diagnosis—case studies.
2. Tuberculosis, Pulmonary—therapy—case studies.   WF 300 S346t 1995]
RC312.2.S35   1995
616.9′95—dc20
DNLM/DLC
for Library of Congress   95-25187
                                                                         CIP

TUBERCULOSIS PEARLS   ISBN 1-56053-156-8

Library of Congress catalog card number 95-25187.

Last digit is the print number: 9 8 7 6 5 4 3 2 1

DEDICATION

This book is dedicated to the patients of the Bellevue Chest Service.

THE PEARLS SERIES®

Series Editors

Steven A. Sahn, M.D.
Professor of Medicine
Director, Division of Pulmonary
and Critical Care Medicine
Medical University of South
Carolina
Charleston, South Carolina

John E. Heffner, M.D.
Professor of Clinical Medicine
University of Arizona
Health Sciences Center
Chairman, Academic Internal Medicine
St. Joseph's Hospital and Medical Center
Phoenix, Arizona

The books in The Pearls Series® contain 75–100 case presentations that provide valuable information that is not readily available in standard textbooks. The problem-oriented approach is ideal for self-study and for board review. A brief clinical vignette is presented, including physical examination and laboratory findings, accompanied by a radiograph, EKG, or other pertinent illustration. The reader is encouraged to consider a differential diagnosis and formulate a plan for diagnosis and treatment. The subsequent page discloses the diagnosis, followed by a discussion of the case, clinical pearls, and two or three key references.

CARDIOLOGY PEARLS
Blase A. Carabello, MD, William L. Ballard, MD, and **Peter C. Gazes, MD,** Medical University of South Carolina, Charleston, South Carolina
1994/233 pages/illustrated/ISBN 0-932883-96-6

CRITICAL CARE PEARLS
Steven A. Sahn, MD, Medical University of South Carolina, Charleston, South Carolina, and **John E. Heffner, MD,** St. Joseph's Hospital and Medical Center, Phoenix, Arizona
1989/300 pages/illustrated/ISBN 0-932883-24-9

INTERNAL MEDICINE PEARLS
Clay B. Marsh, MD, and **Ernest L. Mazzaferri, MD,** The Ohio State University College of Medicine, Columbus, Ohio
1992/300 pages/90 illustrations/ISBN 1-56053-024-3

PULMONARY PEARLS
Steven A. Sahn, MD, Medical University of South Carolina, Charleston, South Carolina, and **John E. Heffner, MD,** St. Joseph's Hospital and Medical Center, Phoenix, Arizona
1988/250 pages/illustrated/ISBN 0-932883-16-8

PULMONARY PEARLS II
Steven A. Sahn, MD, Medical University of South Carolina, Charleston, South Carolina, and **John E. Heffner, MD,** St. Joseph's Hospital and Medical Center, Phoenix, Arizona
1995/300 pages/illustrated/ISBN 1-56053-121-5

TUBERCULOSIS PEARLS
Neil W. Schluger, MD, and **Timothy J. Harkin, MD,** Bellevue Hospital and NYU Medical Center, New York, New York
1996/220 pages/illustrated/ISBN 1-56053-156-8

CONTENTS

Patient	Page

FOREWORD

Tuberculosis has been the most extensive, lethal illness of humankind over the past 250 years. In the 20th century it has receded as a result of improved socioeconomic and housing conditions, curative medications, widespread use of BCG vaccine, and—perhaps—the natural waning of an epidemic infection. But, with the advent of HIV infection/AIDS, tuberculosis is again poised to defend its title as the "The Captain of All These Men of Death."

In the United States, tuberculosis has been and remains a disease with disproportionate impact on immigrants and minorities. And, New York City, the major conduit through which come "your tired, your poor, your huddled masses yearning to breathe free. . ."* has borne a major portion of America's tuberculosis burden.

The Chest Service at Bellevue Hospital has been a bulwark of tuberculosis care in New York City over the past century, led by such inspiring clinician scientists and teachers as J. Burns Amberson, Julia Jones, and John McClement. The proud tradition is carried on today under the leadership of William Rom and colleagues, including those who authored this creative text.

This series of clinical vignettes is filled with cases laden with valuable lessons regarding diagnosis, treatment, prevention, and public health control of tuberculosis. Analogous to the Harvard Law School "Case-Teaching" system, this method is a highly effective and memorable means of conveying vital information for students of this remarkably complex and subtle disease. These "pearls" are the real things.

Michael D. Iseman, M.D.
Chief, Clinical Mycobacterial Service
National Jewish Center for Immunology
    and Respiratory Medicine
Professor of Medicine
University of Colorado School of Medicine
Denver, Colorado

---

*Emma Lazarus: The New Colossus: Inscription for the Statue of Liberty, New York Harbor.

EDITORS' FOREWORD

In all ages, physicians have delighted in solving challenging clinical problems. Not only do patients benefit from a well-directed diagnostic approach, but clinicians experience a unique sense of professional satisfaction when years of experience pry open a diagnostic dilemma.

The Pearls Series® is directed toward this aspect of the physician's nature. In editing these books, we have attempted to develop a consistent format and style that challenge the reader with the salient features of a clinical problem and direct attention to an important question in management. The discussion that follows first reviews the patient's general disorder and then focuses on the unique aspects of the presented patient's condition. Throughout the discussion, aspects of diagnosis and care that are especially important, "cutting edge," or not widely recognized are captured and listed at the end of the text as "Clinical Pearls." Finally, so as not to lose sight of our interest in the individual patient, the discussion closes with the clinical outcome of the patient at hand. In the process, student readers beginning their medical careers, residents in training, and experienced clinicians honing their skills will find something of value in each of the patient presentations.

We compliment Drs. Neil Schluger and Timothy Harkin, who join the list of Pearls authors, for their superb accomplishment in bringing together such a broad array of clinical problems related to the diagnosis and management of tuberculosis. This topic has re-emerged as one of the most important public health issues of our decade. We hope that this text serves as a practical resource and trustworthy guide to assist physicians in the care of these patients.

John E. Heffner, M.D.
Steven A. Sahn, M.D.
Editors, The Pearls Series®

PREFACE

Tuberculosis is an ancient disease that maintains an importance today that can be stated simply: it is the leading cause of death of adults due to infection in the world. The cases presented in this text represent patients seen on the Bellevue Hospital Chest Service over the past few years, and are thus demonstrative of the continuing challenges posed by tuberculosis. Our own interest in tuberculosis stems not only from the fascinating clinical aspects of the disease, but also from the intertwined relationship between the medical and social aspects of tuberculosis. To study the history of tuberculosis through the ages is in a very real sense to study the history of all of medicine and society at large. In the present day, one cannot understand tuberculosis without understanding the epidemiology and immunology of AIDS, social conditions in urban areas in the United States and around the world, the politics and funding of public health programs, behavioral aspects of adherence to medical regimens, and the human host response to infection. The cases in this volume address all these issues and many more.

The cases presented here have been culled from the records of the Bellevue Chest Service. The Chest Service was founded in 1903 by James Alexander Miller, and was the first inpatient hospital unit in the United States dedicated to the care of patients with tuberculosis. That mission is still a major focus of the Chest Service today. In its 93-year history, the Bellevue Chest Service has been led by only five individuals: James Alexander Miller, J. Burns Amberson, John McClement, H. William Harris, and the current chief, William N. Rom, M.D., M.P.H. These men have maintained a dedication not only to the clinical care of patients with tuberculosis but also to the advancement of knowledge of fundamental clinical and basic science issues related to tuberculosis. Their legacy inspired us as we wrote this book.

In 1920 Marcus Sinclair Patterson, then the superintendent of the Brompton Hospital Sanatorium, wrote that the eradication of tuberculosis "will demand a mobilization of all forces, medical as well as social, and even then it will prove a great and difficult problem." We hope that with this volume we have made a small contribution to that effort, and we hope that readers will find it useful in the care and management of their patients with tuberculosis.

Neil W. Schluger, M.D.
Timothy J. Harkin, M.D.

ACKNOWLEDGMENTS

We wish to thank Georgeann McGuiness, M.D., David P. Naidich, M.D., and Robert Lawrence, M.D. for their help in obtaining the radiographs and identifying some of the cases used in this volume. We also thank William N. Rom, M.D., M.P.H., Chief of the Bellevue Chest Service and Director of the Division of Pulmonary and Critical Care Medicine of the New York University Medical Center, for his advice and encouragement throughout this project.

We consider ourselves fortunate to have learned much of what we know about tuberculosis from H. William Harris, M.D., a master teacher and clinician.

We are forever grateful to Linda Belfus for her guidance, good humor, and support throughout this project, and to our editors, Drs. John Heffner and Steven Sahn, who demonstrated extraordinary patience, skill, and encouragement.

PATIENT 1

A 48-year-old man with a pulmonary infiltrate, a positive tuberculin test, and negative sputum smears

A 48-year-old man presented with a 10-week history of a nonproductive cough. He otherwise felt well, denying fever, chills, night sweats, weight loss, or dyspnea. The patient smoked one pack of cigarettes per day for the last 25 years, worked as a cook, and denied drug or alcohol abuse as well as HIV risk factors.

Physical Examination: Afebrile. General: healthy appearing. Chest: clear to auscultation and percussion. Cardiac: normal.

Laboratory Findings: Hct 42%; WBC 8,900/μl. Electrolytes and liver function tests: normal. Tuberculin skin test: 20-mm induration. Chest radiograph: bilateral upper lobe nodular infiltrates (shown below). Sputum acid-fast stains: three negative induced specimens. Sputum cultures: negative for mycobacteria. HIV test: negative.

Question: How should this patient be managed?

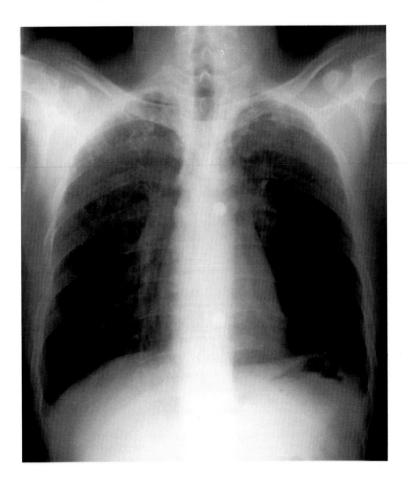

Diagnosis: Smear-negative, culture-negative pulmonary tuberculosis.

Discussion: Many patients with a positive tuberculin test and radiographic evidence of active tuberculosis have negative sputum smears and cultures for acid-fast bacilli. Sputum smears are relatively insensitive for the detection of mycobacterial organisms. Approximately 5,000–10,000 organisms per ml of sputum must be present for the acid-fast stain to be positive. Sputum smears are more likely to be positive, therefore, in patients with cavitary disease who have a heavy bacillary load. Sputum cultures are more sensitive than smears, but are negative in about one-fifth of patients with active pulmonary tuberculosis.

The management of suspected tuberculosis in the setting of negative sputum smears and cultures depends on the likelihood that the patient actually has tuberculosis as well as the consequences of a mistaken empiric diagnosis. Patients from areas with a high prevalence of tuberculosis who have radiographic evidence of active disease and no history of previous antituberculous therapy have a high clinical likelihood of tuberculosis regardless of the sputum findings. The presence of a negative tuberculin skin test result does not greatly decrease the likelihood of active disease. Established practice, therefore, has been to initiate empiric therapy in such patients on presentation because of the long wait for culture results. Although clinical practice is no doubt in evolution due to the potential of greater diagnostic certainty offered by bronchoscopy and the potential of more rapid culture results offered by radiometric techniques, empiric therapy remains a valid and important treatment option.

Recent clinical studies support this empiric approach. Thirty-five percent of patients who had four negative smears at initiation of four-drug antituberculosis therapy in a study from Hong Kong (a high prevalence region for tuberculosis) eventually had positive cultures. In a study from Arkansas (another high tuberculosis prevalence region), a similar proportion of patients who had negative sputum smears and cultures had radiographic or clinical evidence of a response to therapy, confirming the correctness of empiric therapy in these patients. In fact, both studies found that 4 months of multidrug therapy led to relapse rates of 1% to 4% in smear-negative patients, which is comparable to relapse rates in smear-positive patients who receive 6 months of drug treatment. These findings have led to the current recommendations that patients with radiographic findings compatible with tuberculosis and a positive tuberculin test at ≥ 5 mm receive only 4 months of multidrug therapy if they are smear- and culture-negative.

Patients with HIV disease and suspected tuberculosis, however, represent a special clinical group. These patients typically have varied radiographic manifestations of tuberculosis that cannot be easily diagnosed on clinical grounds alone. Additionally, other complications of AIDS may simulate manifestations of tuberculosis and progress rapidly if not diagnosed early and treated correctly. Recommendations for empiric antituberculous therapy for suspected tuberculosis do not apply to patients with HIV disease.

The present patient was treated with a 4-month course of a multidrug regimen of antituberculous drugs and had a progressive improvement in the cough and pulmonary infiltrates.

Clinical Pearls

1. Culture-negative tuberculosis accounts for about 15% of all cases of tuberculosis. Patients with symptoms and radiographic findings consistent with tuberculosis should be considered candidates for chemotherapy even if cultures are negative.

2. In cases of culture-negative tuberculosis, symptomatic improvement and radiographic resolution of findings are the guide to therapy.

3. Four months of chemotherapy may be acceptable for patients with radiographic findings compatible with tuberculosis and a positive tuberculin test of ≥ 5 mm.

REFERENCES

1. Hong Kong Chest Service/British Medical Research Council. A controlled trial of 2-month, 3-month, and 12-month regimens of chemotherapy for sputum-smear-negative pulmonary tuberculosis: results at 60 months. Am Rev Respir Dis 1984;130:23–28.
2. Dutt AK, Moers D, Stead WW. Smear- and culture-negative pulmonary: four-month short-course chemotherapy. Am Rev Respir Dis 1989;139:867–870.
3. Hong Kong Chest Service/Tuberculosis Research Centre, Madras/British Medical Research Council. A controlled trial of 3-month, 4-month, and 6-month regimens of chemotherapy for sputum-smear-negative pulmonary tuberculosis: results at 5 years. Am Rev Respir Dis 1989;139:871–876.

PATIENT 2

A 30-year-old man with active pulmonary tuberculosis

A 30-year-old man with a history of alcoholism presented with a 3-week history of fever and a cough productive of green sputum. He also smoked cigarettes but denied other known medical problems.

Physical Examination: Temperature 101.3°F, pulse 76, respirations 16, blood pressure 130/76. General: thin, chronically ill-appearing. HEENT: normal. Chest: diminished breath sounds at the right apex and at the left base. Cardiac: normal heart sounds without murmurs or rubs. Abdomen: normal. Neurologic: normal.

Laboratory Findings: Hct 40%, WBC 7,800/μl. Electrolytes, liver function tests, coagulation profile: normal. Chest radiograph: diffuse infiltrates. A sputum smear was positive for acid-fast bacilli.

Question: What therapy should be instituted for this patient?

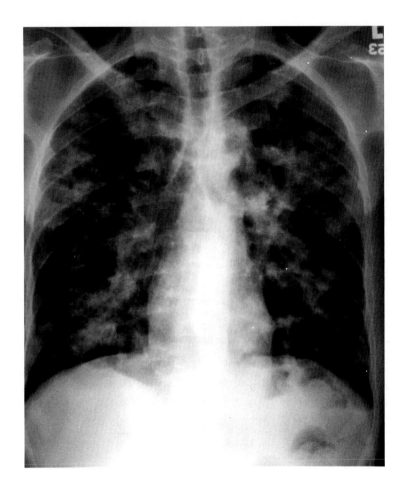

Diagnosis: Pulmonary tuberculosis.

Discussion: Although several different drug combinations and therapeutic regimens are effective in the management of tuberculosis, they all rely on the same fundamental principles. The cornerstone of these principles is the initiation of multidrug therapy to prevent the emergence of resistant pathogens. Several combination regimens presently exist that effectively achieve bacteriologic cure with acceptably low rates of relapse.

The current recommendations of the American Thoracic Society and the Centers for Disease Control offer three potential regimens for initial treatment.

1. Daily isoniazid, rifampin, pyrazinamide for 8 weeks followed by 16 weeks of isoniazid given either daily or twice or thrice weekly. In areas where the rate of isoniazid resistance is known to be greater than 4%, ethambutol or streptomycin must be added to the initial regimen.

2. Daily isoniazid, rifampin, pyrazinamide, and either streptomycin or ethambutol for 2 weeks followed by 6 more weeks of the four drugs given twice weekly, and then followed by 16 more weeks of isoniazid and rifampin given twice weekly.

3. Thrice weekly isoniazid, rifampin, pyrazinamide, and ethambutol or streptomycin for 6 months.

In addition, a 9-month regimen consisting solely of isoniazid and rifampin given daily is an acceptable regimen but should generally be reserved for situations in which other drugs cannot be used or are not tolerated.

With all of the above regimens, there are several important caveats. First, before instituting any antituberculous chemotherapy, a complete history of prior treatment and susceptibility testing results on previously isolated acid-fast organisms must be obtained. If there is any question of drug-resistant tuberculosis, none of the above regimens may be appropriate for initial therapy and an expert in management of tuberculosis should be consulted. Second, all intermittently administered regimens must be given in a setting of directly observed therapy (DOT) to guarantee patient compliance. Third, all drug regimens should be reassessed when drug susceptibility results become available. The above regimens are acceptable only for fully sensitive strains of tuberculosis. Fourth, if sputum smears remain positive or if the patient remains symptomatic after 3 months of therapy, the treating physician should seek the advice of an expert in the care of patients with tuberculosis. A single agent should never be added to a failing antituberculous regimen.

In addition to the above caveats, there may be other circumstances in which the above regimens may not be suitable for initial empiric therapy. For example, pregnant patients should not be treated with regimens that contain pyrazinamide or streptomycin. Also, patients with active tuberculosis who were close contacts of individuals with multidrug-resistant tuberculosis need specialized regimens to ensure adequacy of therapy.

The present patient was started on a regimen of isoniazid, rifampin, pyrazinamide, and ethambutol, in consideration of the greater than 4% rate of isoniazid resistance in New York City.

Clinical Pearls

1. Multi-agent chemotherapy is the cornerstone of any effective short-course regimen.

2. A thorough history of prior treatment and drug susceptibility testing results should be obtained in patients with previous tuberculosis before reinstituting therapy.

3. All-short course, intermittent regimens must be administered in the setting of directly observed therapy.

4. Patients should be reevaluated by experts in tuberculosis therapy if no clinical improvement or conversion of sputum cultures to negative occurs after 3 months of therapy.

REFERENCES

1. Johnston RF, Wildrick KH. The impact of chemotherapy in the care of patients with tuberculosis. Am Rev Respir Dis 1974;109:636–664.
2. Combs DL, O'Brien RJ, Geiter LJ. USPHS tuberculosis short course therapy trial 21: effectiveness, toxicity, and acceptability. The report of final results. Ann Intern Med 1990;112:397–406.
3. Cohn DL Catlin BJ, Peterson KL, et al. A 62-dose, 6-month therapy for pulmonary and extrapulmonary tuberculosis. Ann Intern Med 1990;112:407–415.
4. American Thoracic Society. Treatment of tuberculosis and tuberculosis infection in adults and children. Am J Respir Crit Care Med 1994;149:1359–1374.

PATIENT 3

A 41-year-old man with tuberculosis and noncompliance with medical therapy

A 41-year-old man with a known history of active pulmonary tuberculosis and HIV infection presented with fever, chills, and a productive cough. He had been admitted to another hospital 2 weeks previously, where a diagnosis of sputum-smear-positive pulmonary tuberculosis was established. The patient was not presently on antituberculous drug therapy.

Physical Examination: Temperature 104.5°F, respirations 20, pulse 88, blood pressure 120/80. General: ill-appearing man. Head: normal. Neck: shotty cervical adenopathy. Chest: diminished breath sounds over the left lower and mid-lung fields. Heart: normal heart sounds without murmurs. Abdomen: normal. Extremities: normal. Neurologic: normal.

Laboratory Findings: Hct 25%, WBC 5,900/μl. Na$^+$ 129 mEq/L, K$^+$ 3.9 mEq/L, Cl$^-$ 101 mEq/L, HCO$_3^-$ 21 mEq/L. ABG (room air): pH 7.38, PaCO$_2$ 37 mmHg, PaO$_2$ 78 mmHg. Liver function tests: AST (SGOT) 192 IU/L. Chest radiograph (shown below): cavitary infiltrate in the left upper lobe, adenopathy in the aorto-pulmonary window. Sputum examination: positive for acid-fast bacilli.

Questions: What treatment should be instituted? What infection control measures should be taken to protect hospital staff and other patients from infection?

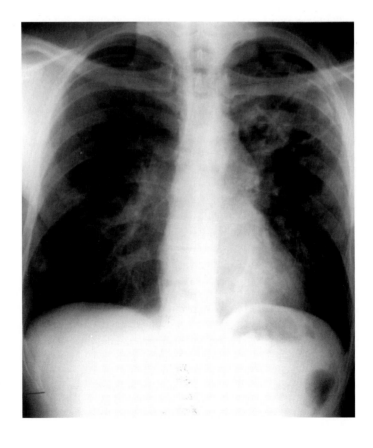

Diagnosis: Smear-positive pulmonary tuberculosis.

Discussion: Clinicians may in certain instances decide to hospitalize a patient with smear-positive tuberculosis in order to protect potential contacts from exposure to the disease. Co-morbidity from other illnesses, such as HIV infection, or social factors, such as a lack of stable housing, often provide additional compelling reasons for hospital admission. Hospitalization of extremely infectious patients, however, may actually create a greater exposure risk to more individuals than what would have occurred if the patient had remained in the community. Nosocomial outbreaks of tuberculosis have been reported to occur when patients with unusual presentations of tuberculosis or extrapulmonary disease were admitted with unrecognized disease. Unfortunately, many outbreaks have been reported in which patients with straightforward presentations of pulmonary tuberculosis or known disease were managed on wards or in ICUs without appropriate infection control measures. These reports emphasize the importance of implementing effective strategies to prevent the nosocomial transmission of tuberculosis to staff and other patients.

Factors that correlate with a high infectiousness include the presence of radiographic evidence of cavitary disease, positive sputum smears, laryngeal tuberculosis, pronounced cough, and the absence of appropriate drug therapy. Because tuberculosis is spread by respiratory droplet nuclei, a patient with only extrapulmonary disease is not likely to be infectious. Recognition of these clinical features associated with infectiousness is the first component of any successful infection control program, as clearly the unsuspected or unknown case of tuberculosis is much more dangerous than one that is clearly identified. When a patient with suspected tuberculosis is identified, a series of hierarchical infection control measures should be instituted, consisting of administrative, environmental, and personal (respiratory mask) components.

At the administrative level, hospital areas at high risk for tuberculosis transmission should be identified. These areas usually include the emergency department and outpatient clinic areas, as well as procedure rooms, such as operating rooms and bronchoscopy suites. Staff working in these areas should be educated to recognize possible cases of tuberculosis early so that patients can be urgently triaged and placed in appropriate isolation.

Effective isolation requires the coordination of the three available environmental infection control procedures available. These three procedures have varying amounts of evidence supporting their efficacy and include modified ventilation, ultraviolet germicidal radiation, and air filtration. Reasonably good data support modified ventilation and the concept that constant introduction of fresh air into a room dilutes the number of infectious particles in the environment. A standard of six air exchanges per hour, therefore, is included in government recommendations for tuberculosis control. Implementation and maintenance of systems necessary for this air exchange, however, entail considerable expense. Germicidal ultraviolet radiation is a potentially cheaper means of cleansing the air and can be combined with high-volume air flow systems, which theoretically yield the equivalent of 12–15 air exchanges per hour. Ventilation and ultraviolet radiation have at times been combined with high-efficiency filtration, though the added effect of this component is difficult to assess.

Great controversy has arisen over personal respiratory protection using tight-fitting particulate respirator masks. The masks are uncomfortable, expensive, and may not provide protection in situations where protection is needed most. These masks may be most appropriate for extremely high-risk situations, such as bronchoscopy suites, where procedures are performed on high-risk subjects.

Once a patient with suspected tuberculosis is admitted, every effort should be made to quickly establish the diagnosis and to institute proper therapy. This requires a laboratory capable of rapid turnaround for sputum smears with reliable results. Once a patient has been started on therapy, isolation is usually continued until sputum smears are negative on 3 consecutive days. Upon discharge, some mechanism to guarantee completion of treatment, such as a program of directly observed therapy, is mandatory. The safest tuberculosis patient is one who is being correctly treated with an effective drug regimen.

The present patient was kept in isolation in the emergency department until a ward bed was available. He was later transferred to an isolation room that had ultraviolet light sources, six air exchanges per hour, and negative pressure ventilation. He was treated with isonizid, rifampin, pyrazinamide, and ethambutol and kept in isolation until sputum smears were negative on three successive examinations. He was discharged with his medications given by directly observed therapy.

Clinical Pearls

1. The first level of infection control for tuberculosis involves educating staff in high-risk areas to maintain a high level of suspicion for detecting patients with active tuberculosis.

2. Administrative (triage, isolation) and environmental controls are more important than personal respiratory protection for limiting the nosocomial transmission of tuberculosis.

3. Infection control does not stop upon discharge. Physicians must take steps to ensure compliance with therapy after a patient leaves the hospital.

REFERENCES

1. Riley R, Nardell EA. Clearing the air: the theory and application of ultraviolet air disinfection. Am Rev Respir Dis 1989; 139:1286–1294.
2. Centers for Disease Control. Guidelines for preventing the transmission of tuberculosis in health-care settings, with special focus on HIV-related issues. MMWR 1990;39:1–29.
3. Iseman MD. A leap of faith. What can we do to curtail intrainstitutional transmission of tuberculosis? Ann Intern Med 1992;117:251–253.
4. Adal KA, Anglim AM, Palumbo CL, et al. The use of high-efficiency particulate air-filter respirators to protect hospital workers from tuberculosis: a cost-effectiveness analysis. N Engl J Med 1994;331:169–173.
5. Nettleman MD, Fredrickson M, Good NL, Hunter SA. Tuberculosis control strategies: the cost of particulate respirators. Ann Intern Med 1994;121:37–40.
6. Jarvis WR, Bolyard EA, Bozzi CJ, et al. Respirators, recommendations, and regulations: the controversy surrounding protection of health care workers from tuberculosis. Ann Intern Med 1995;122:142–146.
7. Maloney SA, Pearson ML, Gordon MT, et al. Efficacy of control measures in preventing nosocomial transmission of multidrug-resistant tuberculosis to patients and health care workers. Ann Intern Med 1995;122:90–95.

PATIENT 4

A 33-year-old hospital worker with a positive tuberculin skin test

A 33-year-old man from Mexico was examined in the hospital's employee health service for a routine yearly evaluation and tuberculin skin test. The patient was employed as a morgue worker. He was generally healthy without complaints or known exposures to tuberculosis. The patient had no risk factors for HIV infection.

Physical Examination: Vital signs: normal. General: comfortable. Head: normal. Chest: normal. Heart: normal heart sounds without murmurs or rubs. Abdomen: normal. Extremities: normal. Neurologic: normal.

Laboratory Findings: CBC, electrolytes, liver function tests: normal. Tuberculin skin test: 15 mm of induration. Chest radiograph (shown below): normal.

Questions: How should this patient's positive tuberculin test be evaluated? Is treatment with isoniazid preventive therapy indicated without disease in a high-risk individual?

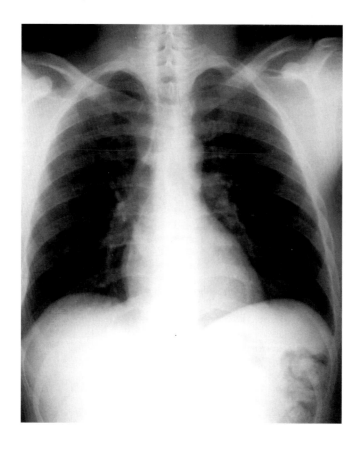

Diagnosis: Tuberculosis infection without active disease in a high-risk individual.

Discussion: The decision to institute isoniazid chemoprophylaxis is made by weighing the risks and benefits of therapy. Specifically, the benefit to the patient is the reduction in likelihood of active tuberculosis in the future. The risk to the patient is the possibility of developing chemical hepatitis from isoniazid. Isoniazid-induced hepatitis is usually reversible, but may be severe and life-threatening in some patients.

It is estimated that in otherwise healthy persons with asymptomatic tuberculosis infection, the lifetime risk of developing active tuberculosis ranges from 5–10%. The majority of risk occurs in the first few years after acquiring the infection. The risk increases with certain underlying diseases or conditions, such as silicosis, chronic renal failure, postgastrectomy states, malnutrition, malignancy, prolonged immunosuppressive therapy, and diabetes. Underlying HIV disease creates the greatest risk, with AIDS patients having a 10% chance *per year* of developing active tuberculosis. Diabetics are at the low end of the risk spectrum, with perhaps a two times risk of reactivating their disease compared to completely healthy persons.

Other factors, such as the patient's occupation, may play a role in decision making. A health care worker or an individual working in a congregate setting, such as a group home or homeless shelter, may place many vulnerable persons at risk if he or she develops active tuberculosis. It is recommended to institute isoniazid preventive therapy in such persons, and even to screen them at intervals as frequent as every 6 months.

Weighing against institution of isoniazid chemoprophylaxis is the chance of developing a serious complication of the therapy. Although minor side effects, such as a pruritic skin rash, are common but easily managed, severe and occasionally fulminant hepatitis is the most dreaded complication of therapy. Transient, asymptomatic increases in liver function tests are common in patients receiving prophylactic isoniazid, and are generally of no consequence. However, potentially life-threatening hepatitis has been estimated to occur in 1 in 10,000 cases, and the incidence of this severe complication rises considerably after age 35. Isoniazid preventive therapy, therefore, is not recommended after age 35 unless the patient has a very high risk of developing active tuberculosis.

A recent analysis, however, indicated that the risk of severe isoniazid hepatitis may be overestimated. This analysis was based on a review of published literature and public health records and estimated that the rate of fatal isoniazid hepatitis was 0.001% (2 in 202,497 patients) overall and 0.002% (1 in 43,334) in persons over age 35. This study and its methodology have not been repeated or validated in other populations.

Current ATS recommendations are to obtain baseline liver function tests in all patients about to begin isoniazid. If the tests are normal at baseline, patients under 35 years of age can be monitored clinically, but patients over 35 require monthly liver function tests.

The ATS recommends the institution of isoniazid chemoprophylaxis when a tuberculin test is positive for patients with or at risk for HIV infection, close contacts of patients with newly diagnosed tuberculosis, recent tuberculin skin test converters, persons with other medical conditions that increase the chance of developing active tuberculosis, persons under age 35 from high prevalence countries or medically underserved areas, or residents of long-term care facilities or institutions. Persons without any risk factor under age 35 with a positive tuberculin reaction of 15 mm or greater are also candidates for preventive therapy. For all others except HIV-infected persons, the cutoff is a tuberculin reaction of 10 mm. In HIV-infected persons, 5 mm of induration defines a positive test.

The present patient should have received isoniazid prophylaxis on several counts: he was under 35 years of age with >15 mm of induration, he worked in a health care facility, and he came from a high-risk country. The radiographic finding of right hilar calcification was not in itself an indication for preventive therapy, but it did dispel any potential doubts regarding the true positivity of the tuberculin test result. Unfortunately, the treating physician did not initiate chemoprophylaxis and the patient developed active pulmonary tuberculosis 2 years later.

Clinical Pearls

1. The decision to institute isoniazid chemoprophylaxis should be made after consideration of the risks and benefits of therapy to the patient.

2. An otherwise healthy adult with a positive tuberculin skin test has a 5–10% lifetime risk of developing active tuberculosis.

3. Recent data suggest that the risk of severe isoniazid-induced hepatitis in adults older than 35 years of age is lower than previously reported, occurring in fewer than 1 in 40,000 patients.

REFERENCES

1. Fitzgerald JM, Gafni A. A cost-effectiveness analysis of the routine use of isoniazid prophylaxis in patients with a positive Mantoux skin test. Am Rev Respir Dis 1990; 142: 848–853.
2. Salpeter SR. Fatal isoniazid-induced hepatitis: its risk during chemoprophylaxis. West J Med 1993;159:560–564.
3. American Thoracic Society. Treatment of tuberculosis and tuberculosis infection in adults and children. Am J Respir Crit Care Med 1994;149:1359–1375.

PATIENT 5

A 29-year-old man from China with pulmonary tuberculosis

A 29-year-old man presented to the hospital complaining of fever and cough of 5 months' duration. He had emigrated from China 9 months earlier. There was no history of previous tuberculin skin testing, and the patient denied close contact with any person with tuberculosis. He worked in a clothing factory. There was no significant past medical history.

Physical Examination: Temperature: 104°F. General: no acute distress. Chest: diminished breath sounds over the right upper lung field. Heart: normal heart sounds without murmurs. Abdomen: normal. Extremities: normal. Neurologic: normal.

Laboratory Findings: Hct 38%, WBC 8,300/μl. Serum electrolytes, liver function tests, coagulation profile: normal. Chest radiograph (shown below): infiltrates in the right upper and right middle lobes. Sputum examination: positive for acid-fast bacilli.

Questions: What is the diagnosis? What special measures need be taken, if any, considering the patient's background?

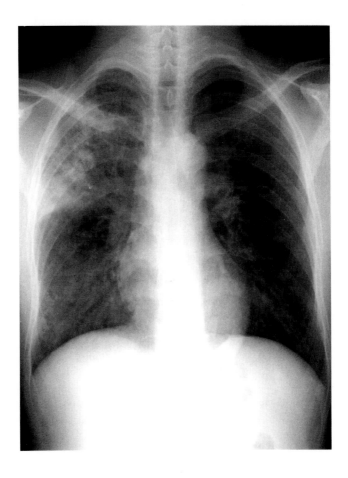

Diagnosis: Pulmonary tuberculosis in a recent immigrant from China.

Discussion: The World Health Organization (WHO) classifies tuberculosis as the leading cause of death due to infectious disease in the world, with over 15 million new cases and at least 3 million deaths yearly. The highest incidence of cases is in the developing world, including areas of South America, sub-Saharan Africa, and Asia, where prevalence rates can be higher than 200 cases per 100,000 persons. This is in contrast to a prevalence of approximately 10/100,000 persons in the United States and 15–20/100,000 in most of Western Europe (although Portugal has a rate closer to 60/100,000). The consequences of these high prevalence rates around the world are several. First, it is unlikely that tuberculosis will be eradicated as a global problem in the forseeable future, because countries with the highest prevalence rates have little resources to spend on diagnosis and treatment. This fact, coupled with the lack of an effective vaccine, ensures the importance of tuberculosis as a health threat into the 21st century.

The contribution of foreign-born persons to the total number of cases of tuberculosis in the United States varies predictably with immigration patterns in different regions of the country. In New York City, foreign-born persons contribute about one-quarter of the total case load of tuberculosis. In San Francisco, however, foreign-born persons account for slightly over half of all cases. These data emphasize the importance of screening high-risk populations for asymptomatic tuberculous infection. Data are available from several programs in the United States and Canada, and they indicate that while tuberculin screening of unselected populations is not an effective public health measure, targeting of certain groups can be an effective tuberculosis control strategy.

Despite foreign-born persons being an obvious high-risk group, several barriers to effective tuberculosis control remain. First, language constitutes an important hurdle. There is a dearth of both persons with the needed language skills and lay literature that can provide information to the wide variety of immigrant groups that exist in the United States. Second, fears about the government may cause immigrants to avoid contact with the public health authorities. Third, fear of stigmatization or of being returned to the country of origin because of ill health may keep patients away from doctors. Fourth, many foreign-born persons use traditional health practices in preference to Western medical care. It is not uncommon in New York City, for example, to see patients who have been treated by herbalists for months for their tuberculosis before

seeking medical attention in a hospital or clinic. Herbal medicine may provide temporary relief of symptoms for some patients, as these preparations are often laced with corticosteroids. Physicians must be sensitive to all of these issues when reaching out to communities of foreign-born persons at risk for tuberculosis.

The Centers for Disease Control estimates that the incidence of tuberculosis among persons entering the United States is 124/100,000, or nearly 10 times the rate for the United States as a whole. Most of these cases develop within 5 years of immigration to this country. A study from Denver Department of Health screened 7,573 recent immigrants (nearly all from Mexico) for tuberculosis infection and found that 42% of evaluable cases were tuberculin skin test positive, using a 10-mm cutoff. The incidence of tuberculin positivity was 36% among people from Europe and Canada, 43% from Mexico, and 58% of those from South America. The cohort of persons screened consisted largely of persons between the ages of 15 and 35 years. Using widely accepted criteria for institution of isoniazid preventive therapy, treatment was recommended for 1,029 people. Interestingly, only 16 cases of active tuberculosis were discovered in the screening process. The cost of this program was estimated to be roughly $3,000 per case of tuberculosis prevented, a figure that compares well to the cost of treating an active case.

A study of Asian immigrants to Canada found that although active tuberculosis was diagnosed in very few persons who were screened for disease, the incidence of active disease in the years following arrival was eight times higher in the immigrants than for native Canadians. This again points out the opportunity for reduction in the case rate by the use of tuberculin screening programs and the application of isoniazid preventive therapy.

Current recommendations of the United States Advisory Committee for Elimination of Tuberculosis are that all persons applying for permanent entry into the United States be screened for disease, and that tuberculin skin testing and preventive therapy programs for foreign-born persons should be expanded overseas and domestically.

The present patient had active pulmonary tuberculosis and was initiated on a four-drug regimen because of the likelihood of resistant pathogens acquired in China. Sputum culture results identified the presence of pan-sensitive organisms. Review of his immigration records showed that he had not been properly screened for tuberculosis.

Clinical Pearls

1. Foreign-born persons from countries with a high prevalence of tuberculosis should be screened both for active disease and infection when permanently moving to a low prevalence country.

2. An aggressive approach to isoniazid preventive therapy should be taken with persons from high-incidence countries.

3. Screening for tuberculosis infection will be an extremely effective measure for reducing active tuberculosis cases in certain regions of the United States where foreign-born individuals account for a substantial proportion of cases.

REFERENCES

1. Centers for Disease Control. Tuberculosis among foreign-born persons entering the United States. Recommendations of the Advisory Committee for Elimination of Tuberculosis. MMWR. 1990;39:(RR-18):1–21.
2. Wang JS, Allen EA, Enarson DA, Grzybowski S. Tuberculosis in recent Asian immigrants to British Columbia, Canada: 1982–1985. Tubercle 1991;72:277–283.
3. Blum RN, Polish LB, Tapy JM, et al. Results of screening for tuberculosis in foreign-born persons applying for adjustment of immigration status. Chest 1993;103:1670–1674.
4. Capobianco DJ, Brazias PW, Fox TP. Proximal-muscle weakness induced by herbs. N Engl J Med 1993;329:1430.

PATIENT 6

A 41-year-old man with an abnormal chest radiograph and negative sputum acid-fast bacilli smears

A 41-year-old man presented with complaints of fever and night sweats. He had a history of recent incarceration and use of crack cocaine but denied intravenous drug use. His PPD skin test had been noted to be positive several years earlier, but he had never been treated with isoniazid preventive therapy. The patient had no history of active tuberculosis.

Physical Examination: Temperature: 100.6°F, remainder of vital signs: normal. General: no acute distress. Head: normal. Chest: few crackles at the left apex. Heart: normal heart sounds without murmurs; Abdomen: normal. Neurologic: normal.

Laboratory Findings: CBC and electrolytes: normal. HIV antibody: negative. Chest radiograph (shown below): left apical infiltrate. Microscopic examination of sputum samples (collected on three successive days): negative for acid-fast organisms.

Questions: What is the likely diagnosis? How should the patient be managed?

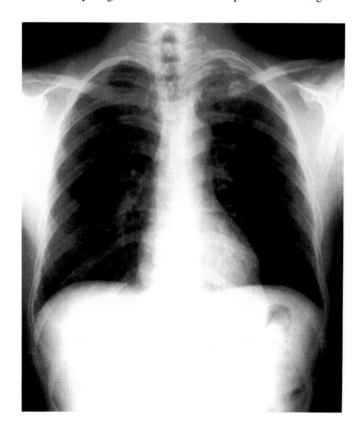

Diagnosis: Active, smear-negative pulmonary tuberculosis.

Discussion: The patient with smear-negative, active pulmonary tuberculosis presents a challenging clinical problem. Proper management depends on a clear understanding of the relative yields of different diagnostic tests in a variety of clinical settings.

Sputum examination remains the most rapid approach to the diagnosis of pulmonary tuberculosis. In most areas of the country, a positive sputum examination indicates a high probability of *M. tuberculosis* infection. Other conditions that may present with positive acid-fast smears include infections with atypical mycobacteria, nocardia, and some legionella species that may be (usually weakly) acid-fast. The sensitivity of sputum examination, however, is only 50–75%. Certain clinical characteristics seem to be associated with higher rates of positive sputum smears, such as the presence of cavitary le- sions on chest radiographs. When tuberculosis appears clinically likely, however, a negative sputum smear can never exclude the presence of active disease.

In the absence of positive sputum smears, the clinician evaluating a patient with suspected tuberculosis can choose several diagnostic approaches. A reasonable choice in many instances is to institute empiric multidrug antituberculous therapy pending culture results. This approach is appropriate if the clinical index of suspicion for active tuberculosis is high and the differential diagnosis seems limited. If cultures are positive, therapy can be continued and adjusted for antibiotic susceptibility. If cultures are negative, patients can be continued on therapy and considered to have culture-negative tuberculosis if they demonstrated a clinical and radiographic response to therapy. Patients failing to respond require further diagnostic evaluations.

If considerable diagnostic uncertainty exists at initial presentation of a patient with suspected tuberculosis who has negative smears, it may be appropriate to pursue a more aggressive diagnostic investigation. Unfortunately, bronchoscopy remains the only option to expectorated sputum examination to achieve a more prompt clinical diagnosis of pulmonary tuberculosis. Several retrospective studies of the utility of fiberoptic bronchoscopy in the diagnosis of tuberculosis have been done, and although each study has its limitations, it is possible to draw general conclusions. Most studies indicate that the immediate diagnostic yield from bronchoscopy in patients with smear-negative active disease is in the range of 40%. The largest and best designed studies indicate that the diagnostic yield of bronchoalveolar lavage alone for diagnosis is almost negligible. Transbronchial biopsy with demonstration of granuloma, acid-fast bacilli, or both has the highest yield for an immediate diagnosis. For this reason, most centers always perform transbronchial biopsy for suspected tuberculosis.

Because of the infectious risks to the operators, however, bronchoscopy should be reserved for instances in which considerable diagnostic uncertainty exists. Extreme attention should be paid to the problem of occupational risk of tuberculosis in this era of multidrug-resistant organisms. One should always bear in mind that failure to demonstrate granulomata or acid-fast bacilli on bronchoscopy specimens in no way rules out the diagnosis of active pulmonary tuberculosis.

Because the chest radiograph of the present patient was characteristic of active pulmonary tuberculosis, he was empirically treated with a four-drug regimen of isoniazid, rifampin, ethambutol, and pyrazinamide. Six weeks later, sputum cultures grew *M. tuberculosis,* confirming the clinical diagnosis.

Clinical Pearls

1. Up to 50% of patients with active pulmonary tuberculosis have negative sputum smears.

2. Empiric therapy for tuberculosis is a reasonable alternative for a large proportion of patients with suspected tuberculosis. Revisions to therapy can be made after final culture results and clinical response are evaluated.

3. If fiberoptic bronchoscopy is performed in an attempt to diagnose tuberculosis, transbronchial biopsy is an important component of the procedure. Negative results from bronchoscopy do not exclude active tuberculosis as a diagnostic possibility.

REFERENCES

1. Gordin FM, Slutkin G, Schecter G, et al. Presumptive diagnosis and treatment of pulmonary tuberculosis based on radiographic findings. Am Rev Respir Dis 1989;139:1090–1093.
2. Kennedy DJ, Lewis WP, Barnes PJ. Yield of bronchoscopy for the diagnosis of tuberculosis in patients with human immunodeficiency virus infection. Chest 1992;102:1040–1044.
3. Schluger N, Rom WN. Current approaches to the diagnosis of active pulmonary tuberculosis. Am J Respir Crit Care Med 1994;149:264–267.

PATIENT 7

A 7-year-old girl with a right middle lobe infiltrate

A 7-year-old girl was admitted with 1 week of cough productive of yellow sputum and fever. One month earlier, a tuberculin test placed during a school physical examination was noted to be positive. Although the patient was referred to a physician who ordered a chest radiograph that showed right hilar adenopathy, she was not started on any therapy. Her fever and cough began 3 weeks later. There was no known contact with anyone with active tuberculosis, although the girl's parents were also tuberculin test positive.

Physical Examination: Temperature 104°F, pulse 110, respirations 25, blood pressure 106/68. General: acutely ill-appearing girl. Head: normal. Chest: rhonchi in right mid-lung field. Heart: normal. Abdomen: normal. Extremities: normal. Neurologic: normal.

Laboratory Findings: Hct 32%, WBC 25,000/μl. Serum electrolytes and liver function tests: normal. Chest radiograph (shown below): right mid-lung infiltrate. Sputum smear: negative for acid-fast bacilli.

Questions: What is the diagnosis? What therapy should be instituted?

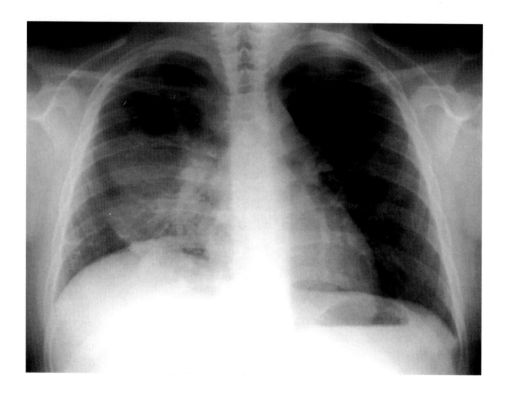

Diagnosis: Primary tuberculosis.

Discussion: Pediatric tuberculosis remains a global problem, with the pediatric population contributing about one-sixth of the total cases worldwide. The recent increase in the prevalence of tuberculosis in adults in the United States has been paralleled by a similar rise in pediatric cases. This association is not surprising considering that almost all children who become infected with tuberculosis have been exposed to an adult with infectious disease. The adult sources cases are usually a member of the child's household. The younger the child, the less likely that a child with tuberculosis contracted the disease from outside of the household. Therefore, prevention of tuberculosis in children depends on identifying and treating adults with active tuberculosis who live with children.

The risk that a child will develop active tuberculosis after infection, as well as the severity of disease, is related to the age of the child. Approximately 70% of all children with tuberculosis are less than 5 years old, and this age group is at increased risk for miliary disease and meningitis. In comparison to a 10% lifetime risk of developing active disease after infection for an adult, infants have a 50% risk, while children between 1 and 5 years old have a 25% risk.

The risk that a child will infect others with tuberculosis is also related to age. Children who are less than 10 years old are rarely infectious for a number of reasons. Children tend to have a lower incidence of cavitary lung disease, a lower bacillary burden, and a less forceful cough than adults, thus leading to a much lower number of organisms shed in expelled sputum. Furthermore, about 25% of children have extrapulmonary tuberculosis, which is typically noninfectious.

The manifestations of tuberculosis in children reflect the relatively rapid progression from infection to active, primary disease. Miliary disease is the most common form in infants and children coinfected with HIV. In older children, bulky lymphadenopathy with compression of bronchi and endobronchial involvement, or progressive primary tuberculosis with cavities not in the typical apical location are common. The most frequent extrapulmonary forms in children are lymphadenitis in up to 60%, especially in the head and neck, and meningitis, which occurs in about 10–15%. Manifestations more characteristic of reactivation of infection are generally not seen until the adolescent years.

Congenital tuberculosis is a rare but often deadly occurrence. Infection may occur transplacentally by the hematogenous route, or by ingestion of infected amniotic fluid during birth. Disease becomes apparent by the second or third week, but tuberculosis is rarely suspected unless the mother is known to have active tuberculosis. Almost one-half of cases are diagnosed at postmortem examination.

The same factors that make children with tuberculosis less infectious than adults make the diagnosis more difficult to confirm, as sputum specimens containing organisms are rarely obtainable. To take advantage of swallowed respiratory secretions that may contain mycobacteria, smears and cultures of aspirated gastric contents are usually collected. At best, about 5% of smears and 40% of cultures of gastric aspirates will be positive. Cultures obtained from involved extrapulmonary sites may also be helpful. Radiographic findings of intrathoracic adenopathy or a miliary pattern, either by standard chest radiograph or chest CT, are suggestive of tuberculosis. However, about 50% of cases of pediatric tuberculosis are diagnosed without bacteriologic confirmation.

In general, treatment strategies for active tuberculosis in children are similar to those employed in adult patients. The frequent lack of positive cultures means that susceptibility patterns of the organisms are usually not available to help guide therapy. Therefore, every effort should be made to identify the source case that infected a child in order to obtain the susceptibility pattern of the adult's organism that can guide the treatment of the child. If the organism from the source case is known to be sensitive to isoniazid and rifampin, or if the source case cannot be identified, the child should be treated with standard short-course therapy. Isoniazid (10–15 mg/kg), rifampin (10–20 mg/kg), pyrazinamide (20–25 mg/kg), and ethambutol (15 mg/kg) should be administered daily, preferably through a directly observed therapy program. Using the ethambutol dose of 15 mg/kg, the complication of retrobulbar neuritis should occur in less than 1% of patients. Nonetheless, caution should be exercised in the use of this medication in children whose visual acuity cannot be assessed; some clinicians advocate substitution of another drug, such as an aminoglycoside, in this setting. In the treatment of children with drug-resistant tuberculosis, the use of quinolones may be necessary. The long-term use of quinolones in children is of concern, however, because these agents cause limb abnormalities in dogs in utero. Despite this concern, clinical use of the quinolones in children thus far has been safe, but further investigation in this area is needed. The addition of steroids to antituberculous therapy should be considered in the setting of compressive lymphadenopathy causing bronchial obstruction, and in meningitis with evidence of cranial nerve involvement.

The current patient was started on a standard four-drug regimen of isoniazid, rifampin, pyrazinamide, and ethambutol, as no source case could be identified. Her sputum cultures subsequently grew *M. tuberculosis* sensitive to all agents. Her symptoms rapidly responded to treatment.

Clinical Pearls

1. The manifestations of tuberculosis in children are usually those of primary disease, reflecting recent infection from an adult source case.

2. Children with tuberculosis are usually not infectious because of a lower incidence of cavitary lung disease, lower bacillary burden, less forceful cough, and a higher incidence of extrapulmonary disease.

3. Less than 50% of children with tuberculosis will have bacteriologic confirmation of disease, so treatment is usually empiric and should be guided by the drug susceptibilities of the source case, when available.

4. The theoretic concern of retrobulbar neuritis in children receiving ethambutol whose visual acuity cannot be assessed should not preclude its use at a dose of 15 mg/kg/day when indicated.

REFERENCES

1. Starke JR, Jacobs RF, Jereb J. Resurgence of tuberculosis in children. J Pediatr 1992;120:839–855.
2. American Academy of Pediatrics, Committee on Infectious Diseases. Chemotherapy for tuberculosis in infants and children. Pediatrics 1992;89:161–165.
3. Abadco DL, Steiner P. Gastric lavage is better than bronchoalveolar lavage for isolation of *Mycobacterium tuberculosis* in childhood pulmonary tuberculosis. Pediatr Infect Dis 1992;11:735–738.
4. Bakshi SS, Alvarez D, Hilfer DL, et al. Tuberculosis in human immunodeficiency virus-infected children: a family infection. Am J Dis Child 1993;147:320–324.

PATIENT 8

A 39-year-old man with dyspnea and a miliary pattern on chest radiograph

A 39-year-old man presented with progressive shortness of breath. Four days earlier, he had been seen at another hospital's emergency department for this complaint. The patient was told that his chest radiograph was abnormal, but he chose not to be further evaluated. He denied fever, chills, sweats, weight loss, or cough. There was no other significant history.

Physical Examination: Vital signs: normal. General: comfortable. HEENT: normal. Chest: fine bibasilar crackles. Cardiac: normal heart sounds, without murmurs or rubs. Abdomen: normal. Extremities: normal. Neurologic: normal.

Laboratory Findings: Hct 34%, WBC 5,600/μl. Electrolytes, liver function tests, and coagulation profile: normal. Tuberculin skin test: negative. Chest radiograph (closeup views shown below): diffuse small nodules. Sputum smear: negative for acid-fast bacilli.

Question: What diagnostic procedures should be done to confirm the diagnosis in this patient?

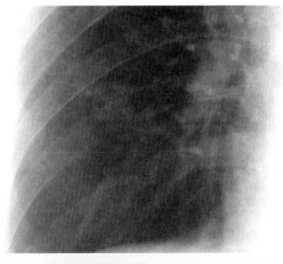

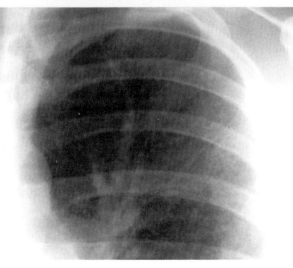

Diagnosis: Miliary tuberculosis.

Discussion: The appearance on a chest radiograph of multiple (far too many to count) small nodules distributed throughout all lung fields suggests the diagnosis of miliary tuberculosis. Classically, miliary nodules are 1–2 mm in diameter and signify that hematogenous dissemination of mycobacteria has occurred throughout the circulation. Dissemination can occur either as a manifestation of primary infection or during reactivation of latent disease.

The age distribution and clinical presentation of miliary tuberculosis vary depending on the clinical setting and the presence of comorbid conditions. A recent study from South Africa noted that 8.3% of children (mean age of presentation 10.5 months) and only 1.3% of adults with tuberculosis had miliary disease. In other studies, the effects of underlying HIV disease has been examined in adults with miliary tuberculosis. These studies indicate that patients without AIDS present with miliary tuberculosis at a mean age of 60 years, have comorbid conditions in two-thirds of instances, and experience a 21% mortality. Patients with AIDS tend to be younger and often demonstrate cutaneous anergy and more severe degrees of anemia, leukopenia, and thrombocytopenia. The mortality of miliary tuberculosis in patients with AIDS is 25%.

Even though the miliary lesions on the chest radiograph are the most clinically apparent manifestations of the disease, patients with miliary tuberculosis have mycobacteria and resulting granuloma formations in multiple organs throughout the body. Manifestations of this dissemination is often nonspecific, but specific symptoms can localize to nearly any organ system. Similarly, laboratory studies are often abnormal but nonspecific. The presence of anemia is especially common. Tuberculin skin tests are less often positive in miliary tuberculosis than in other forms of the disease. Patients are also less likely to have positive sputum smears for acid-fast bacilli; the diagnostic yield of this study is as low as 25–50%. Sputum cultures, however, may be positive in as many as two-thirds of patients.

The differential diagnosis of a miliary pattern on a chest radiograph includes a broad array of infections and malignancies that can disseminate hematogenously. Histoplasmosis, particularly in patients with AIDS, *Pneumocystis carinii* pneumonia, and hematogenous spread of carcinoma of the thyroid are the most common conditions that simulate the radiographic appearance of miliary tuberculosis. Although the diagnosis of miliary tuberculosis can be strongly suspected from the chest radiograph, a definitive diagnosis depends on demonstration of the characteristic histopathology of granulomata and culture of mycobacteria. Chest CT scans demonstrate that the miliary lesions in the lungs result from granulomata distributed randomly in the pulmonary interstitium. Because these nodules may have sharp or poorly defined borders on CT, this examination is rarely diagnostic of the disorder.

In confirming the diagnosis, biopsy specimens are usually obtained from the lung, liver, or bone marrow. Tissues obtained from these sites generally have a diagnostic yield greater that 85%. Many experts recommend selecting an initial site of biopsy on the basis of the most prominent clinical finding. For instance, a patient with an abnormal chest radiograph without other localizing signs or symptoms would be selected for bronchoscopy with transbronchial biopsy. This procedure will also allow the exclusion of other diagnostic possibilities, such as histoplasmosis. For patients with miliary tuberculosis and negative sputum smears, bronchoscopy can provide a diagnosis in 83% of patients, which is a higher diagnostic yield than in other sputum-smear-negative forms of pulmonary tuberculosis. Patients with a normal chest radiograph or a nondiagnostic transbronchial biopsy might undergo a bone marrow biopsy if peripheral blood abnormalities are prominent findings. In any event, liver biopsy is usually reserved for later in the diagnostic evaluation because of the greater morbidity attached to this procedure.

Current recommendations for treating miliary tuberculosis are the same as for any other form of the disease.

On the basis of his clinical presentation and abnormal chest radiograph, the present patient was suspected to have miliary tuberculosis. He underwent fiberoptic bronchoscopy with a transbronchial biopsy that demonstrated granulomata. Sputum cultures subsequently grew *Mycobacterium tuberculosis*. He was treated with a standard antituberculosis regimen with good results.

Clinical Pearls

1. Miliary tuberculosis can represent either primary infection or reactivation with hematogenous spread.

2. Sputum smears have a much lower yield in miliary compared to other forms of pulmonary tuberculosis; a negative smear should not dissuade the clinician from pursuing the diagnosis in the proper clinical setting.

3. Biopsy of lung, liver, and bone marrow all have high diagnostic yields, but in cases in which the disease is clinically confined to the lungs, fiberoptic bronchoscopy provides the most direct route to diagnosis.

4. Treatment is the same for miliary tuberculosis as for other forms of pulmonary tuberculosis.

REFERENCES

1. Sahn SA, Levin DE. The diagnosis of miliary tuberculosis by transbronchial lung biopsy. Br Med J 1975;2:667–668.
2. Willcox PA, Potgieter PD, Bateman ED, Benatar SR. Rapid diagnosis of sputum negative miliary tuberculosis using the flexible fibreoptic bronchoscope. Thorax 1986;41:681–684.
3. Kim JH, Langston AA, Gallis HA. Miliary tuberculosis: epidemiology, clinical manifestations, diagnosis, and outcome. Rev Infect Dis 1990;12:583–590.
4. Maartens G, Willcox PA, Benatar SR. Miliary tuberculosis: rapid diagnosis, hematologic abnormalities, and outcome in 109 treated adults. Am J Med 1990;89:291–296.
5. Hill AR, Premkumar S, Brustein S, et al. Disseminated tuberculosis in the acquired immunodeficiency syndrome era. Am Rev Respir Dis 1991;144:1164–1170.
6. McGuiness G, Naidich DP, Jagirdar J, et al. High resolution CT findings in miliary lung disease. J Comp Assist Tomogr 1992;16:384–390.

PATIENT 9

A 40-year-old woman with an abnormal chest radiograph and sputum positive for *M. tuberculosis* by the polymerase chain reaction

A 40-year-old woman with a history of smoking presented for evaluation of an abnormal chest radiograph. She complained of malaise but denied fever, chills, or cough. The patient was bisexual but had never been tested for HIV. She stated that a tuberculin test performed 1 year previously had been negative.

Physical Examination: Temperature 102.6°F, pulse 100, respirations 18 and blood pressure 106/74. General: thin, comfortable. HEENT: 1-cm rubbery left anterior cervical lymph node. Chest: normal. The remainder of the examination was normal.

Laboratory Findings: Hct 34%, WBC 3,400/μl. Electrolytes and liver function tests: normal. Chest radiograph (shown below): large right paratracheal mass. Sputum AFB smear: negative. Polymerase chain reaction assay of sputum: positive for DNA of *M. tuberculosis*. HIV antibody testing: refused.

Question: What is the significance of the polymerase chain reaction result in this patient?

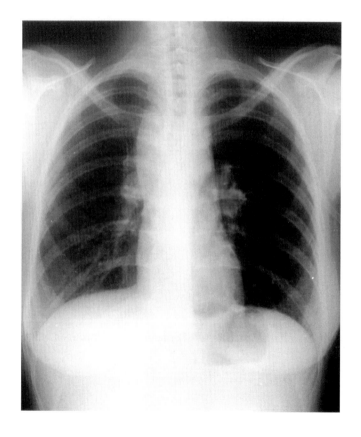

Diagnosis: The results support the diagnosis of mediastinal tuberculous lymphadenitis.

Discussion: One of the most exciting developments in laboratory diagnostics in the past several years has been the polymerase chain reaction (PCR) assay. PCR is a method of DNA amplification that can detect the presence of DNA from a single cell. This technology potentially offers an unmatched ability to determine the presence of minute amounts of genetic material. The application of PCR technology to the diagnosis of infectious diseases has great potential; however, the precise role of this technology in clinical medicine is yet to be determined.

The principle of the PCR assay is simple. Small fragments of DNA (primers) that are synthesized in the laboratory are added to the DNA that has been extracted from a clinical specimen, such as sputum, pleural fluid, blood, or bone marrow. If the DNA sequences of the primers match the DNA in the clinical specimen, the primers will bind to that DNA and millions of identical copies of the target DNA of interest can be synthesized. Such large amounts of DNA can be easily detected with standard electrophoresis techniques. To apply the technique to the diagnosis of tuberculosis, primers are used that recognize a DNA sequence (called IS6110) unique to the *M. tuberculosis* complex of organisms. If no *M. tuberculosis* DNA is present in the sample to which the primers are added, no amplification will take place. However, if even a few *M. tuberculosis* organisms are present (orders of magnitude fewer than would be required for a positive smear or culture), they will be detected easily. Other mycobacterial species, such as *M. avium, kansasii, fortuitum,* will not be detected with the *M. tuberculosis*-specific primers.

Clinical experience with the PCR assay for diagnosis of tuberculosis has been limited to date. It has been shown that essentially all smear-positive cases of tuberculosis are accompanied by a positive sputum PCR result. However, there has been limited experience in evaluating the assay in the situation where it could have the greatest utility—smear-negative, culture-positive tuberculosis. In a series of 65 patients with suspected tuberculosis, of whom 12 were smear-negative and culture-positive, all 12 had *M. tuberculosis* DNA detected in their sputum using PCR analysis. In the same study, however, several positive PCR results on sputum were found in patients who had only a remote history of tuberculosis or a positive tuberculin skin test with a normal chest radiograph. It may be that the PCR assay is too sensitive, and that in some patients a positive result may indicate the residue of prior or quiescent infection.

Recently, the PCR assay has been applied to DNA extracted from peripheral blood monocytes of patients with pulmonary tuberculosis. Investigators found that DNA from *M. tuberculosis* could be detected in the peripheral blood (buffy coat fraction) of all eight patients they tested with culture-proven, active pulmonary tuberculosis. Healthy tuberculin-positive and tuberculin-negative controls did not have evidence of circulating mycobacterial DNA. This intriguing preliminary finding warrants continued investigation.

Although PCR is one of the most promising new developments in the diagnosis of tuberculosis, its precise clinical role remains to be determined, especially in smear negative cases.

The present patient had a transbronchial needle aspiration biopsy of the paratracheal mass that yielded acid-fast bacilli. Subsequent cultures for *M. tuberculosis* were positive, thereby confirming the PCR result.

Clinical Pearls

1. The polymerase chain reaction assay can detect DNA from as few as one organism in a variety of biologic samples.

2. PCR can rapidly confirm that acid-fast organisms in a specimen belong to the *M. tuberculosis* complex (*M. tuberculosis, M. microti, M. africanum, and M. bovis*), and can distinguish these organisms from any other mycobacterial species.

3. The precise clinical role of PCR remains to be determined, particularly when the test is applied to patients with previously treated tuberculosis.

REFERENCES

1. Eisenach KD, Sifford MD, Cave MD, et al. Detection of *Mycobacterium tuberculosis* in sputum samples using a polymerase chain reaction. Am Rev Respir Dis 1991;144:1160–1163.
2. Schluger NW, Kinney D, Harkin TJ, Rom WN. The clinical utility of the polymerase chain reaction in the diagnosis of infections due to *Mycobacterium tuberculosis*. Chest 1994;105:1116–1121.
3. Schluger NW, Condos R, Lewis S, Rom WN. Amplification of DNA of *Mycobacterium tuberculosis* from peripheral blood of patients with pulmonary tuberculosis. Lancet 1994; 344: 232–233.

PATIENT 10

A 30-year-old prisoner with a left upper lobe infiltrate

A 30-year-old man was referred from the local jail because of an abnormal chest radiograph that was obtained during routine screening after his arrest. The patient reported a 3-month history of weight loss, night sweats, and an occasionally productive cough. This was his fifth arrest in the past 5 years, but he had not been incarcerated for more than 6 months at a time. His past medical history was significant for syphilis and gonorrhea. He denied risk factors for HIV but admitted smoking cocaine.

Physical Examination: Temperature 101.8°F. Chest: bronchial breath sounds and egophony left upper lobe.

Laboratory Findings: CBC and electrolytes: normal. Chest radiograph: left upper lobe infiltrate. Sputum: positive for acid-fast bacilli.

Question: What risks for disease need to be considered when evaluating prisoners?

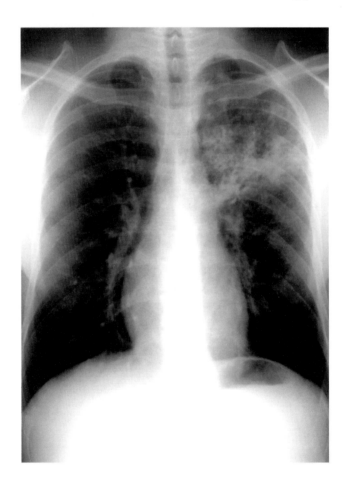

Diagnosis: Pulmonary tuberculosis.

Discussion: Infection control measures to limit the risks of nosocomial tuberculosis in acute care hospitals present hospital epidemiologists with major challenges. Prevention of the spread of tuberculosis in other types of facilities presents even greater challenges that vary on the basis of the institution's population, as well as the physical design of the institution itself.

Jails have long been recognized as facilities in which the institutional spread of tuberculosis represents a particular risk. A recent study of inmates in a New York City jail demonstrated that the risk of contracting tuberculosis increases with the number of times an inmate enters jail (i.e., the number of re-arrests). This risk most likely results from the placement of large groups of recently arrested prisoners, some of whom have tuberculosis, into a common holding pen before adequate screening for active tuberculosis can be performed. The more times an inmate enters such a holding area, the more likely he or she is to become infected. Length of time spent in jail is also a significant risk factor for infection.

The high rate of recidivism in this population represents an important risk to the communities from which the prisoners come and to which they return after release. Furthermore, the increase in the prevalence of HIV infection among inmates has had a dramatic impact on the spread of tuberculosis within correctional facilities, as illustrated by a recently reported outbreak of multidrug-resistant tuberculosis in a New York State correctional facility.

Shelters for the homeless in major urban areas represent another institution in which a high risk exists for the spread of tuberculosis. Plagued by overcrowded conditions and poor ventilation, shelters house individuals who have a high backround prevalence of tuberculosis based on socioeconomic status. The resulting environment simulates conditions in developing countries where tuberculosis is rampant. It is not surprising, therefore, that shelters in the United States represent unfortunately efficient sites for the spread of tuberculosis. A recent study in a large shelter for the homeless in New York City found that at least 79% of the inhabitants showed evidence of infection.

The crowded conditions in shelters may actually increase the risk of tuberculosis by reinfection. Although previous infection with tuberculosis provides a good measure of protection against reinfection, the poor general health of the homeless, malnourishment, substance abuse, and infection with HIV may intersect with a heavy exposure to airborne infectious particles that can overwhelm the natural immunity. Thus exogenous reinfection

followed by active disease has shared blame with reactivation of prior infection for the continuing spread of tuberculosis in shelters.

Nursing homes are also sites where conditions exist for the spread of tuberculosis. Because of their advanced age, many nursing home residents have had ample opportunities to have been remotely infected with tuberculosis. A landmark study of all nursing home inhabitants in Arkansas found that 10–15% of newly admitted residents had positive tuberculin skin tests; almost twice as many inhabitants who had been in the homes for more than a month reacted to tuberculin, demonstrating a high rate of infection during residence in the homes. Subsequent tuberculin testing found that 5% of inhabitants of a nursing home who were in residence with a coresident who had infectious tuberculosis converted to a positive skin test each year. In comparison, only 3.5% of nursing home inhabitants converted each year if there was not an identified coresident with active disease, suggesting a number of unsuspected infectious cases in those homes. Approximately 6% of the new converters who did not receive preventive therapy with isoniazid went on to develop active tuberculosis. Unsuspected active tuberculosis poses a serious potential risk of new infection for nursing home residents.

The nursing home study cited above clearly illustrates the central tenet of prevention of transmission of tuberculosis: priority must be placed on the rapid identification of patients with active, infectious tuberculosis. This must be followed immediately by isolation from others and administration of appropriate treatment. Adherence to this practice is essential to prevent outbreaks within institutional settings. Prisoners and nursing home residents should be screened for tuberculosis with histories, physicals, and tuberculin skin tests. Chest radiographs should be performed in individuals with positive skin tests or other findings suggestive of tuberculosis infection or active disease. Nursing home residents should have two-step skin testing to identify those with tuberculin reactions that have waned. Appropriate treatment for infection or disease should be started, with isolation from the general population as indicated.

To the extent possible when dealing with a transient population, a similar strategy should be employed in shelters for the homeless. As a secondary precaution against infectious patients who have not been identified in prisons and shelters, ulraviolet irradiation and adequate ventilation should be used in common rooms where groups of people are gathered, including holding pens, recreational rooms, and eating halls. These steps will serve to protect uninfected individuals who reside in the institutions, their visitors, the communities to which they may return, as well as those who work in the institutions.

The current patient was placed in a respiratory isolation room. On the basis of his positive sputum sample for acid-fast bacilli, he was started on a standard four-drug regimen. His sputum specimen subsequently grew *M. tuberculosis* sensitive to all drugs.

Clinical Pearls

1. Increased risk of tuberculosis among correctional facility inmates is related to the number of reentries to the prison system after rearrests as well as to the length of stay in the facility.

2. In addition to reactivation of latent infection in an elderly population, reinfection in nursing homes due to undetected or unsuspected cases of active tuberculosis is an important cause of disease in such settings.

3. Decreased immunity in homeless individuals due to poor nutrition, substance abuse, and HIV infection contributes to the importance of reinfection as a source of tuberculosis in shelters.

4. Controlling the spread of tuberculosis in institutions depends on identification, isolation, and treatment of active cases by use of screening with tuberculin skin tests and often chest radiographs, in addition to adjunctive measures such as ultraviolet irradiation and increased ventilation of common rooms.

REFERENCES

1. Stead WW, Lofgren JP, Warren E, Thomas C. Tuberculosis as an endemic and nosocomial infection among the elderly in nursing homes. N Engl J Med 1985;312:1483–1487.
2. Nardell E, McInnis B, Thomas B, Weidhaas S. Exogenous reinfection with tuberculosis in a shelter for the homeless. N Engl J Med 1986;315;1570–1575.
3. Iseman MD. A leap of faith. What can we do to curtail intrainstitutional transmission of tuberculosis? *Ann Intern Med* 1992;117:251–253.
4. Bellin EY, Fletcher DD, Safyer SM. Association of tuberculosis infection with increased time in or admission to the New York City jail system. JAMA 1993;269:2228–2231.
5. Paul EA, et al. Nemesis revisited: tuberculosis infection in a New York City men's shelter. Am J Public Health 1993;83: 1743–1745.

PATIENT 11

A 27-year-old man with cough and a pleural effusion

A 27-year-old man presented with a 2-month history of cough productive of mucoid sputum, fever, and weight loss. He denied hemoptysis. His tuberculin skin test was negative 1 year previously.

Physical Examination: Temperature 101.8°F, respirations 22, pulse 88, blood pressure 110/70. General: thin, no distress. Chest: dull percussion noted, decreased fremitus and diminished breath sounds over the left middle and lower lung fields. Heart: no jugular venous distention, normal heart sounds without gallops or murmurs. Abdomen: normal. Extremities: normal. Neurologic: normal.

Laboratory Findings: Hct 42%, WBC 19,700/µl. Electrolytes, liver function tests: normal. Chest radiograph: massive left-sided effusion. Tuberculin skin test: 12 mm of induration. Pleural biopsy: necrotizing granulomas, without acid-fast organisms.

Questions: What is the presumptive diagnosis? What treatment should be recommended? Should the pleural effusion be drained?

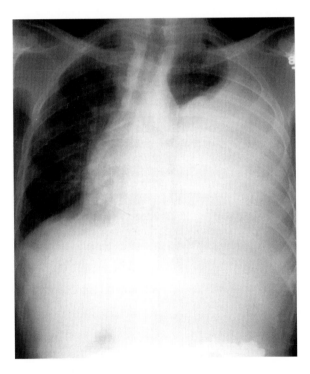

Pleural Fluid Analysis

Appearance: serous

Nucleated cells: 2000/µl

Differential:
  90% lymphocytes
  5% neutrophil
  5% macrophages

RBC: 2500/µl

Total protein: 4.5 g/dl

LDH: 351 IU/L

Glucose: 65 mg/dl

pH: 7.33

Diagnosis: Tuberculous pleurisy.

Discussion: The spectrum of tuberculous infection in the pleural space includes tuberculous pleurisy, tuberculous empyema, bronchopleural fistula, and empyema necessitatis. Each of these conditions has a specific therapeutic approach that may involve antituberculous drug therapy, tube thoracostomy, thoracotomy, and complicated chest wall "thoracoplastic" surgery. Initiation of the correct intervention first requires an understanding of the clinical expression of these various forms of tuberculous pleural disease and the establishment of an accurate clinical diagnosis.

Tuberculous pleurisy can occur during the course of primary tuberculosis 3–6 months after the initial infection or at any time during the life of an untreated, infected patient in the form of reactivation disease. The clinical features of tuberculous pleurisy were first clearly described in a classic patient series collected in the years leading up to but not including the antibiotic era. Sibley reported 200 patients with tuberculous pleural effusions. He found that the onset of symptoms was acute in 163 patients (82%), insidious in 30 (15%), and chronic in 7 (4%). Thirty-seven patients (19%) had no chest pain, but fever and malaise were present in nearly all of the patients. Pleural fluid was most often clear and straw colored, and mycobacteria were grown from 28% of the samples submitted for culture. The yield was greater if large volumes of fluid were cultured.

It was notable in this series that 118 patients (59%) experienced complete or substantial clearing of effusions without the initiation of antituberculous drug therapy. The remainder of patients developed moderate to extensive pleural fibrosis. Normalization of the pleural space occurred more often in patients who were managed with one or more therapeutic aspirations of pleural fluid. Even including the patients who had a seemingly uncomplicated resolution of their pleural effusions, 51% developed active pulmonary or extrapulmonary tuberculosis an average of 10 months after the onset of tuberculous pleurisy. Modern-day patient series confirm the high risk of progressive disease in patients with tuberculous disease, which necessitates the initiation of antituberculous drug therapy in any patient with this disease despite the occurrence of a spontaneous resolution of pleural fluid.

Detection of tubercle bacilli in cultured pleural fluid establishes the diagnosis of tuberculous pleurisy. Unfortunately, only 30% of patients have a positive culture result. Of the available tests, pleural biopsy has the highest diagnostic yield. Up to 75% of patients demonstrate necrotizing granulomas with or without acid-fast organisms when biopsy samples are collected from a single needle insertion site. Up to 90% of patients have positive biopsy results if two separate sites are used. Chest CT may assist the clinical diagnosis in some instances. Many patients with tuberculous pleural effusions have accompanying parenchymal infiltrates suggestive of tuberculosis detected by CT even when the standard chest radiograph fails to demonstrate these lesions.

Once diagnosed, all patients should be treated with standard antituberculous multidrug regimens as recommended by ATS guidelines. When a lymphocyte-predominant, exudative effusion occurs in a patient with a positive tuberculin skin test, antituberculous therapy should be instituted presumptively even if organisms or characteristic histologic changes cannot be detected. The pleural fluid rarely requires drainage, although it is reasonable to drain large to massive tuberculous effusions by thoracentesis to assist in the prevention of progressive pleural fibrosis and a trapped lung. Although corticosteroids have occasionally been used as adjunctive therapy in patients with persistent clinical manifestations of tuberculous pleurisy despite chemotherapy, this form of therapy is rarely required.

Acute tuberculous empyema is an uncommon form of tuberculous pleural disease that occurs from rupture of a parenchymal cavity into the pleural space or the formation of a bronchopleural fistula. Spillage of large numbers of organisms into the pleural space establishes a frank empyema. Well-established parenchymal disease is invariably present. In contrast to simple tuberculous pleurisy, the fluid is purulent, and acid-fast organisms are usually detected on examination of stained specimens. As recommended for nontuberculous causes of empyema thoracis, drainage of the pleural space is mandatory and should be initiated by tube thoracostomy. Surgery may be necessary to close a bronchopleural fistula, which may require extensive chest wall and pleural space manipulation with considerable risk of morbidity and mortality.

Another manifestation of tuberculous infection of the pleural space, empyema necessitatis, occurs as a complication of untreated, chronic tuberculous empyema wherein intrapleural infection dissects through the pleural lining and into the adjacent soft tissue of the chest wall. The pleural fluid usually follows fascial planes, and may track into the vertebral column, retroperitoneum, and paravertebral soft tissues. Chest CT scans demonstrate a thick-walled, well-encapsulated calcified pleural mass associated with an extrapleural mass. The actual fistula track is rarely detected by radiographic examinations. A combined approach with maximum-dose drug therapy and surgical intervention is usually required to manage these patients.

The present patient had classic clinical, radiographic, pleural fluid, and pleural pathologic features of tuberculous pleurisy. He was treated with multidrug short-course antituberculous therapy. His pleural fluid and biopsy sample subsequently grew *M. tuberculosis,* which was sensitive to all first-line antituberculous drugs. The pleural effusion completely resolved during the completion of his drug therapy.

Clinical Pearls

1. The vast majority of patients with tuberculous pleural disease have simple tuberculous pleurisy, which is a hypersensitivity reaction to a small number of organisms in the pleural space. Most patients do not require the addition of repeated needle aspirations, chest tube drainage, or corticosteroids to standard antituberculous drug regimens.

2. Patients with tuberculous empyema require intervention with tube drainage and a thorough search for a bronchopleural fistula.

3. The development of an empyema necessitatis may be the initial clinical manifestation of an underlying chronic tuberculous empyema. These patients usually require extensive resectional surgery to cure their disease.

REFERENCES
1. Sibley JC. A study of 200 cases of tuberculous pleurisy with effusion. Am Rev Tuberc 1950;62:314–323.
3. Bhatt GM, Austin HM. CT demonstration of empyema necessitatis. J Comput Assisted Tomogr 1985;9:1108–1109.
2. Glicklich M, Mendelson DS, Gendal ES, Teirstein AS. Tuberculous empyema necessitatis: computed tomography findings. Clin Imaging 1990;14:23–25.
4. Alzeer AH, FitzGerald JM. Corticosteroids and tuberculosis: risks and use as adjunct therapy. Tuber Lung Dis 1993;74:6–11.

PATIENT 12

A 33-year-old man with HIV disease and a positive sputum culture for *M. tuberculosis*

A 33-year-old man with HIV disease was admitted for evaluation of a positive sputum culture for *Mycobacterium tuberculosis* that was resistant to isoniazid, rifampin, streptomycin, ethambutol, and pyrazinamide. The sputum culture had been obtained for evaluation of a cough (2 months earlier while the patient was in jail). Presently the patient felt well without respiratory complaints. He denied previous opportunistic infections and had no history of known TB exposure.

Physical Examination: Vital signs: normal. General: comfortable. Head: normal. Mouth: no thrush. Neck: no lymphadenopathy. Chest: normal. Cardiac: normal heart sounds, without gallops or rubs. Abdomen: normal. Extremities: normal. Neurologic: normal.

Laboratory Findings: CBC, electrolytes: normal. CD4+ cell count: 300/μl. Tuberculin skin test: negative. Candida and mumps antigen skin tests: reactive. Chest radiograph: normal. Sputum smears for acid-fast organisms: repeatedly negative.

Questions: What is the significance of the sputum culture sent 2 months ago? Does this patient need to be treated?

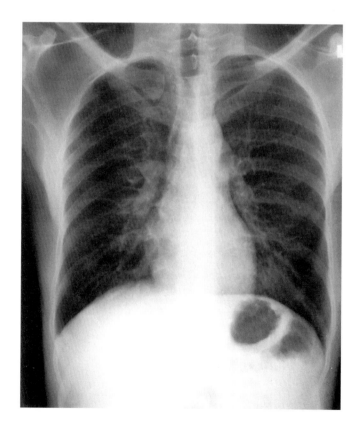

Diagnosis: Primary tuberculosis.

Discussion: A positive sputum culture for *M. tuberculosis* in a patient with a near normal or entirely normal chest radiograph suggests a diagnosis of primary pulmonary tuberculosis. Most patients with this condition present because of respiratory or generalized symptoms and have an abnormal chest radiograph. Occasionally, patients with early primary disease presenting with minor symptoms, such as cough, or high-risk patients undergoing tuberculosis screening may have positive sputum cultures for *M. tuberculosis* and a normal chest radiograph. Indeed, it has been demonstrated that 1–5% of recent close contacts of individuals with active tuberculosis will have positive sputum cultures at a time when the chest radiograph and PPD skin test remain negative.

Patients with primary tuberculosis and a normal chest radiograph may subsequently control their infection or develop progressive primary tuberculosis with the formation of typical radiographic features of the disease. Control of infection may occur through complete elimination of mycobacteria from the lung or containment of viable organisms within granulomata called Ghon complexes. Patients who control their infections typically have low bacterial burdens. Containment of mycobacteria within a Ghon complex is associated with a 10% lifetime risk in normal hosts of developing reactivation tuberculosis. This reactivation risk is markedly reduced by prophylactic therapy with isoniazid. Patients who fail to control their infection and develop progressive primary tuberculosis require therapy with multiple antituberculous drugs.

The coexistence of HIV disease markedly increases the risk of progressive primary tuberculosis and frequently accelerates the course of the disease. Indeed, the high frequency of intrathoracic lymphadenopathy as the presenting radiographic manifestation of tuberculosis in patients with HIV disease indicates the importance of primary compared to reactivation disease in these patients. Furthermore, up to 10% of patients with HIV disease and a positive tuberculosis sputum culture have normal chest radiographs representing early primary disease. In contrast to normal hosts, in patients with HIV disease the risk of development of active tuberculosis and positive sputum mycobacterial cultures despite a normal chest radiograph is 10% *per year*.

Because of the risks of progressive primary tuberculosis, patients with HIV disease and positive sputum cultures for *M. tuberculosis,* despite a normal chest radiograph, should always be treated with multiple drugs as if they already had progressive disease. Even normal hosts with positive sputum cultures despite the absence of symptoms or radiographic abnormalities should be considered for therapy because, unlike other mycobacteria, *M. tuberculosis* is always a pathogen.

The present patient clearly should have been initiated on multi-agent chemotherapy. The primary physicians chose to defer therapy because of his asymptomatic state, normal chest radiograph, and the perceived difficulties in treating multidrug-resistant tuberculosis. Eight months later, fevers and bilateral pulmonary infiltrates developed. Sputum cultures were positive for a strain of *M. tuberculosis* with an identical drug sensitivity profile to the first isolate. Despite initiation of cycloserine, capreomycin, ciprofloxacin, and PAS, he responded poorly and succumbed to his disease.

Clinical Pearls

1. Sputum cultures should not be obtained routinely as a tuberculosis screening measure in general patient populations. Whenever a sputum culture is found to be positive for *M. tuberculosis,* however, therapy should be initiated for presumed disease even if the patient is asymptomatic with a normal chest radiograph.

2. One to 50% of recent close contacts of patients with active tuberculosis will have positive sputum cultures despite having a normal chest radiograph and a negative tuberculin skin test. The skin test will become positive in the overwhelming majority of patients after several weeks.

3. Up to 10% of patients with HIV disease and a positive sputum culture for *M. tuberculosis* will have a normal chest radiograph.

4. The risk of development of active tuberculosis in patients with HIV disease and positive sputum cultures despite normal chest radiograph is 10% per year.

REFERENCES

1. Ward M, Poirer J, Lambert A, et al. Tuberculosis outbreak at a Canadian Forces Base–Ontario. Can Dis Week Rep 1981;7:157.
2. Pedro-Bolet J, Gutiérrez J, Miralles R, et al. Pulmonary tuberculosis in HIV-infected patients with normal chest radiographs. AIDS 1992;6:91–93.
3. Givern MJ, Khan A, Reichman LB. Tuberculosis among patients with AIDS and a control group in an inner-city community. Arch Intern Med 1994;154:640–645.

PATIENT 13

A 44-year-old man with knee pain and an abnormal chest radiograph

A 44-year-old man was admitted to the hospital with right knee pain. The patient, who had immigrated to the United States from China, had an 8-month history of nonspecific inflammatory arthritis involving both knees, for which he had been treated symptomatically with nonsteroidal anti-inflammatory agents. Five days prior to admission, he noted the onset of fever and increased pain and swelling in his right knee. There was no history of trauma to the knee.

Physical Examination: Temperature 102.6°F, other vital signs normal. HEENT: normal, without adenopathy. Chest: clear. Cardiac: normal heart sounds, without murmurs. Abdomen: nontender without organomegaly. Extremities: bilateral knee swelling with effusions; the right knee was tender to palpation, and warm. Neurologic: intact and nonfocal.

Laboratory Findings: CBC and routine serum chemistries: normal. Right knee radiograph: an effusion in the suprapatellar bursa. Chest radiograph: multiple 1–2-mm nodules throughout all lung fields, consistent with miliary tuberculosis. Right knee arthrocentesis: leukocytes 43,000/μl with 73% polymorphonuclear leukocytes. Gram stain of joint fluid: negative, acid-fast stain positive for acid-fast bacilli.

Questions: What are the important considerations in caring for this patient?

Diagnosis: Miliary tuberculosis with tuberculous septic arthritis.

Discussion: The onset of an acute or subacute arthritis in an immunocompromised host should suggest the possibility of tuberculous arthritis. This diagnosis is especially likely in patients with any chest radiographic abnormality compatible with either pulmonary or miliary tuberculosis. The timing of knee complaints in patients with disseminated tuberculosis is interesting in that some patients may have bilateral knee pain for months before the other clinical manifestations of tuberculosis become apparent. This syndrome is called Poncet's disease and may represent an immunologically mediated synovitis akin to the pleuritis that develops in patients with tuberculous pleurisy. Patients with Poncet's disease characteristically progress to clinically active pulmonary or extrapulmonary tuberculosis.

Diagnosing tuberculous arthritis requires consideration of the disease and submission of aspirated synovial fluid for appropriate studies. Direct examination of the fluid with acid-fast stains is positive in 20–30% of patients. Mycobacterial cultures are positive in 60–80% of instances. When patients have tuberculosis arthritis in association with disseminated tuberculosis, which occurs in only 9% of patients, the chest radiograph is often the key to early diagnosis. Up to 6% of immunocompetent hosts and 22% of HIV-infected patients have characteristic "miliary" patterns with 1–2-mm nodules throughout all lung fields that represent granulomata. This pattern represents hematogenous spread of the organism.

Presence of a miliary radiographic pattern indicates a need for urgent diagnosis in that the patient is at risk for rapidly progressive disease and respiratory failure. Examination of sputum smears usually fail to demonstrate acid-fast organisms; sputum cultures are positive, however, in 50–65% of patients. To achieve an early diagnosis, bronchoscopy with transbronchial biopsy is often re-quired. Tissue specimens frequently demonstrate granulomata at least one-third of the time, and cultures of these biopsy samples may be positive. In patients with disseminated disease without chest radiographic abnormalities, biopsy demonstration of granulomata in the bone marrow or liver may confirm the diagnosis. Yields of biopsy from bone marrow or liver are comparable to that of lung, and choice of a site to biopsy often depends on the clinical picture.

Once diagnosed, tuberculous arthritis requires a therapeutic approach that includes antituberculous drugs and consideration of adjuctive surgical care. Patients with low risks of multi-resistant pathogens should receive an initial regimen of isoniazid, rifampin, and pyrazinamide. The duration of therapy for extrapulmonary tuberculous can be 9 months. It is presently uncertain that therapy can be shortened to 6 months. Immunocompetent patients with miliary tuberculosis require only standard antituberculous therapy in the vast majority of cases. Clinical response is the final arbiter of the duration of drug therapy, with clinical response and culture results the most important parameters to follow. Although many patients with tuberculous arthritis were managed with surgical drainage in the past, recent experience indicates that 80% of patients will recover with chemotherapy alone. Surgery is now reserved for patients with extensive bony destruction or progression of disease despite drug therapy.

The present patient appeared to have disseminated tuberculosis on the basis of the miliary chest radiograph, history compatible with Poncet's disease, and positive arthrocentesis result. He was initiated on drug therapy with isoniazid, rifampin, pyrazinamide, and ethambutol, and gradually improved without the need for surgical intervention. After completion of a 9-month regimen of chemotherapy, he was completely asymptomatic with good function of his right knee.

Clinical Pearls

1. The presence of monoarticular arthritis in a patient with any chest radiographic abnormality is compatible with the diagnosis of extrapulmonary tuberculosis.

2. Drug therapy, often accompanied by immobilization, is successful in 80% of patients with tuberculous arthritis.

3. The presence of rheumatic complaints that precede the onset of clinically active tuberculosis is termed "Poncet's disease." Patients with obscure causes of articular complaints should be examined and monitored carefully for the presence of tuberculosis.

REFERENCES

1. Poncet A. De la polyarthrite tuberculeuse deformante or pseudorheumatisme chronique tuberculeux. Congr Fr Chir 1897;2:732–734.
2. Kerri O, Martini M. Tuberculosis of the knee. Int Orthop 1985;9:153–157.
3. Martini M, Ouahes M. Bone and joint tuberculosis: a review of 652 cases. Orthopedics 1988;11:861–866.
4. Dall L, Long L, Stanford J. Poncet's disease: tuberculous rheumatism. Rev Infect Dis 1989;11:105–107.
5. Hodgson SP, Ormerod LP. Ten year experience of bone and joint tuberculosis in Blackburn, 1978–1987. J R Coll Surg Edinb 1990;35:359–362.

PATIENT 14

A 27-year-old pregnant woman with a positive tuberculin test and an abnormal chest radiograph

A 27-year-old woman in her third month of pregnancy presented for evaluation of a positive tuberculin test. The patient was clinically well and denied fever, cough, weight loss, or chest pain. The tuberculin test was performed as part of routine prenatal care. The pregnancy had been completely normal up to that point. The patient was born in Mexico but had lived in the United States for the last 5 years. She had no history of prior tuberculin skin testing, and she denied contact with anyone with active tuberculosis. She had no HIV risk factors.

Physical Examination: Vital signs: normal. General: comfortable. HEENT: normal. Chest: normal. Cardiac: normal. Abdomen: gravid, otherwise normal. Extremities: normal.

Laboratory Findings: CBC, electrolytes, liver functions: normal. Chest radiograph: 1-cm nodular infiltrate/density in the apical segment of the left upper lobe (shown below, arrow). Sputum acid-fast smears: negative.

Question: How should this patient be managed?

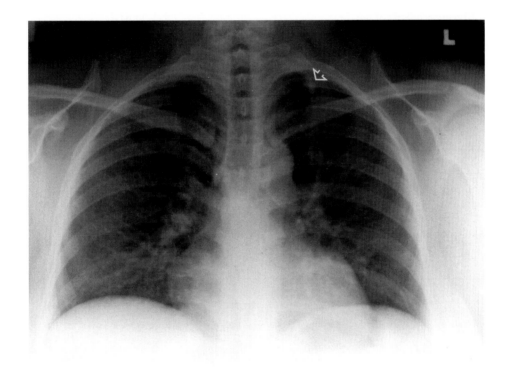

Diagnosis: Calcified granuloma, left upper lobe; tuberculosis infection (inactive).

Discussion: This patient presents a common but vexing clinical problem: the management of a pregnant patient with a positive tuberculin test that may represent either an inactive tuberculosis infection or active disease. To address this problem, pregnant patients with a positive skin test should always undergo a chest radiograph (with abdominal shielding), although it is often appropriate to wait until the second trimester in an asymptomatic patient. If the chest radiograph is normal, the patient is considered for prophylactic therapy with isoniazid. Although there has been fairly widespread experience with isoniazid in pregnancy and the drug is believed to be safe, current recommendations are to defer isoniazid preventive therapy until after delivery unless one of the following conditions is present: the patient is infected with HIV, a close contact of an active case, or a new converter. In all other patients requiring isoniazid prophylaxis, institution of therapy should begin after delivery. New mothers can take isoniazid and continue to nurse, as the levels of isoniazid expressed in breast milk are not toxic to a newborn. However, infants of nursing mothers taking isoniazid should be considered for pyridoxine replacement.

If active tuberculosis is diagnosed during pregnancy, prompt and proper treatment is of great importance both for mother and child. Newborns are extremely susceptible to infection with tuberculosis via the airborne route; true congenital tuberculosis via aspiration of infected amniotic fluid or by hematogenous dissemination through the umbilical cord is quite rare. Untreated mothers who are infectious at the time of delivery pose significant risks to their babies. If the mother is in fact infectious upon delivery, the child may need to be treated and/or removed from the mother for a period of time. Agents that are acceptable for use in treating tuberculosis during pregnancy include isoniazid, rifampin, and most probably ethambutol, although experience with ethambutol is more limited than with the other two. Most authorities believe that the risk of not treating active tuberculosis in pregnancy far outweighs the risks of isoniazid, rifampin, and ethambutol to the fetus. On the other hand, streptomycin and the other aminoglycosides should definitely not be used. No data are available regarding the safety of pyrazinamide in pregnancy, so this agent must be avoided as well. There is little or no information regarding the safety of the second-line agents in pregnancy, so the use of these drugs should be directed in consultation with an expert in the management of drug-resistant tuberculosis.

The present patient was found to have an old chest radiograph taken two years previously. The left upper lobe lesion was present on the earlier radiograph and had not changed in size. The abnormality was considered to be a stable, calcified granuloma, and the patient began isoniazid preventive therapy after delivery.

Clinical Pearls

1. Pregnant women in high-risk groups (including foreign-born persons from high-prevalence countries) should receive tuberculin screening during pregnancy.

2. Positive skin tests must be followed by a complete clinical and radiographic evaluation. Chest radiographs should not be deferred until after delivery.

3. The risks of not treating active or latent tuberculosis in pregnancy are far greater than the risk of antituberculous chemotherapy for the mother or fetus.

REFERENCES
1. McKenzie SA, Macnab AJ, Katz G. Neonatal pyridoxine responsive convulsions due to isoniazid therapy. Arch Dis Child 1976;51:567.
2. Burk JR, Bahar D, Wold FS, et al. Nursery exposure of 528 newborns to a nurse with pulmonary tuberculosis. South Med J 1978;71:7.
3. Good JT, Iseman MD, Davidson PT, et al. Tuberculosis in association with pregnancy. Am J Obstet Gynecol 1981;140:492.
4. Machin GA, Honore LH, Fanning EA, Molesky M. Perinatally acquired neonatal tuberculosis: report of two cases. Pediatr Pathol 1992;12:707–716.
5. Rosenfeld EA, Hageman JR, Yogev R. Tuberculosis of infancy in the 1990s. Pediatr Clin North Am 1993;40:1087–1103.

PATIENT 15

A 52-year-old man with pulmonary infiltrates and positive sputum cultures for
M. kansasii

A 52-year-old homeless man presented with a productive cough, fevers, and a 20-pound weight loss over a 1-year period. Three months earlier, a chest radiograph showed bilateral upper lobe infiltrates with a suggestion of cavitation. At that time, his tuberculin skin test was negative, and multiple sputum smears were negative for acid-fast bacilli. Six of seven sputum cultures, however, grew *M. kansasii*. Before he could be further evaluated, the patient failed to return for subsequent appointments until the current presentation. He denied chills, hemoptysis, and chest pain. He drank 2 quarts of wine per day, took no medications, and smoked a pack of cigarettes a day.

Physical Examination: Temperature 101.2°F. Cardiac: normal. Chest: Bronchial breath sounds and coarse rhonchi over the right upper lobe. Abdomen: normal. Extremities: superficial ulcer of right ankle.

Laboratory Findings: Hct 37%, WBC 6,700/µl. Na$^+$ 130 mEq/l, K$^+$ 3.8 mEq/L, Cl$^-$ 92 mEq/L, HCO$_3^-$ 24 mEq/L. Chest radiograph: shown below. Sputum: positive for rare acid-fast bacilli.

Question: Is further workup of the patient's pulmonary disease necessary?

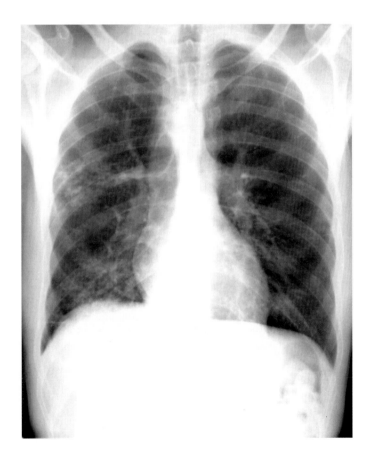

Diagnosis: Pulmonary disease caused by *Mycobacterium kansasii.*

Discussion: M. kansasii and M. avium complex are the two most common nontuberculous mycobacteria to cause human disease. Patients with *M. kansasii* pulmonary infections have many clinical and radiographic similarities with pulmonary tuberculosis, although the clinical manifestations are generally less severe. Extrapulmonary disease and disseminated disease due to *M. kansasii* rarely occur, although dissemination is currently being reported more commonly in patients with AIDS. *M. kansasii* infections occur more commonly in the central United States and have a predilection for white men over the age of 50 who have preexisting lung disease, such as COPD, bronchiectasis, or previous tuberculosis.

As with other nontuberculous mycobacteria, diagnosing *M. kansasii* as the cause of pulmonary disease in an individual patient can be problematic. Skin testing is not helpful and may be confusing, as nontuberculous mycobacteria often cause mildly positive tuberculin reactions, and other species-specific antigens for skin testing are not currently available. A single positive sputum culture for nontuberculous mycobacteria should never be considered diagnostic of disease because these organisms can contaminate culture media and may colonize the airways of patients with chronic lung disease.

Adherence to diagnostic guidelines assist in distinguishing patients with true nontuberculous mycobacterial infections from those who have airway colonization. Radiographic infiltrates or cavities should be present to consider the possibility of infection, and other reasonable causes of these abnormalities should be excluded, including fungal infections, malignancy, and tuberculosis. At least two sputum samples should result in moderate to heavy growth of mycobacteria. In patients with cavities on the chest radiograph (which occurs in up to 90% of patients with disease caused by *M. kansasii,*) these criteria are sufficient to confirm the diagnosis. In patients with noncavitary infiltrates, an additional criterion is imposed: the sputum cultures should remain positive after the initiation of an aggressive bronchial toilet regimen or after 2 weeks of specific antimycobacterial drug therapy. If these criteria are not met in a patient with noncavitary disease and concern remains that nontuberculous mycobacterial disease is present, a biopsy of the abnormal lung should be performed. If a transbronchial, percutaneous, or open lung biopsy specimen shows granulomatous inflammation and culture of the biopsy specimen is positive for *M. kansasii,* a specific diagnosis can be made. If the biopsy specimen demonstrates granulomas but the tissue culture is negative, the combination of light growth of multiple sputum cultures and exclusion of other explanatory diseases is sufficient. In extrapulmonary disease, growth of nontuberculous mycobacteria from a specimen obtained from a normally sterile site is considered diagnostic of disease.

Pulmonary disease due to *M. kansasii* progresses in the absence of therapy, so drug therapy should be started when the diagnosis is established. Patients usually respond well to antituberculous therapy when a rifampin-containing regimen is used. Resistance to rifampin may be acquired, however. Relapse rates are about 1% when a regimen of isoniazid, rifampin, and ethambutol at standard doses is administered for 18 months. If streptomycin at a dose of 1 g two times a week is added for the first 3 months, similar results may be obtained with only 12 months of treatment. If rifampin cannot be used or if resistance is present, bacteriologic and clinical response is slower and relapse rates are in the 10% range. *M. kansasii* is also susceptible to streptomycin, ethionamide, and cycloserine, but is always resistant to pyrazinamide. Standard susceptibility testing is reliable for rifampin, but resistance to low concentrations of isoniazid (≤ 1 mg/ml) or streptomycin (≤ 2 mg/ml) is of no clinical significance and should not lead to an increase in dose when these agents are used.

The present patient met the criteria of heavy growth on multiple sputum cultures and radiographic evidence of cavitary disease for the diagnosis of *M. kansasii* pulmonary infection. He was started on a drug regimen with isoniazid, rifampin, and ethambutol. He refused streptomycin injections. Sputum cultures were negative after 3 months of therapy, and the patient is currently doing well with plans to complete 18 months of treatment.

Clinical Pearls

1. Criteria for diagnosing pulmonary disease due to nontuberculous mycobacteria in the presence of cavitary disease are multiple cultures demonstrating heavy growth and exclusion of other conditions associated with cavitary disease.

2. In the absence of cavities, the additional criterion of failure of sputum culture conversion in response to either aggressive bronchial toilet or 2 weeks of specific antimycobacterial medical therapy needs to be fulfilled.

3. A biopsy specimen of lung revealing granulomata in combination with either a positive biopsy specimen culture or multiple sputum cultures with light growth is also sufficient for diagnosis.

4. Lung disease due to *M. kansasii* should be treated with standard doses of isoniazid, rifampin, and ethambutol for 12 months if streptomycin is given for the first 3 months. Eighteen months of three-drug therapy is indicated if streptomycin is not included in the regimen. The anticipated relapse rate approximates 1%.

REFERENCES

1. Ahn CH, Lowell JR, Ahn SS, et al. Short-course chemotherapy for pulmonary disease caused by *Mycobacterium kansasii*. Am Rev Respir Dis 1983;128:1048–1050.
2. Davidson PT. The diagnosis and management of disease caused by *M. avium* complex, *M. kansasii,* and other mycobacteria. Clin Chest Med 1989;10:431–443.
3. American Thoracic Society. Diagnosis and treatment of disease caused by nontuberculous mycobacteria. Am Rev Respir Dis 1990;142:940–953.

PATIENT 16

A 65-year-old man with diabetes mellitus, a past history of tuberculosis, and a lung mass

A 65-year-old man was referred because of an abnormal preoperative chest radiograph that demonstrated an upper lobe density compatible with lung carcinoma. The patient had a history of diabetes mellitus for several years and was admitted to the hospital for a transmetatarsal amputation of a diabetic foot. There was a history of treated pulmonary tuberculosis 15 years earlier. The patient was a lifelong heavy smoker but denied respiratory symptoms.

Physical Examination: Vital signs: normal. General: healthy appearing. Chest: normal. Cardiac: normal heart sounds, without murmurs or rubs. Abdomen: normal. Extremities: dry gangrene of the left foot.

Laboratory Findings: CBC, electrolytes, and liver function tests: normal. Chest radiograph (shown below): right upper lobe nodular lesion. Fiberoptic bronchoscopy: no endobronchial lesions. Transbronchial biopsy and CT-guided biopsy of the mass: nondiagnostic histopathologic features.

Question: How should the patient be managed?

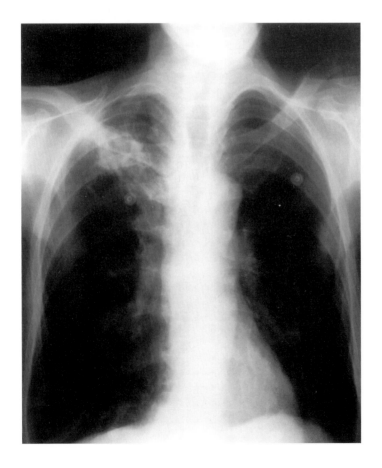

Diagnosis: Reactivation pulmonary tuberculosis presenting as a mass lesion diagnosed by open lung biopsy.

Discussion: Tuberculosis and cancer often mimic each other in their clinical and radiographic presentations. Both disorders frequently produce chronic or subacute symptoms occasionally associated with systemic manifestations such as decreased appetite or weight loss. The radiographic appearance of a solitary pulmonary nodule or multiple nodular lung lesions presents an extensive differential diagnosis within which tuberculosis and lung cancer are prominent disorders.

In approaching a patient with chest radiographic lesions suggestive of either cancer or tuberculosis, not all clinical features assist the clinician in determining the probability of the diagnosis. The absence of symptoms is not helpful, for instance, in patients being evaluated for a solitary pulmonary nodule. In one series of 1000 patients with pulmonary nodules, 75% were asymptomatic, and an equal proportion of these patients had benign versus malignant disease.

The age of the patient, however, can suggest the nature of a solitary pulmonary nodule. Overall, 24% of solitary pulmonary nodules in most reported series are due to tuberculosis, with the highest incidence occurring in younger age populations. Most of the remaining benign causes of lung nodules are fungal granulomas. The proportion of patients with lung cancer is as high as 65% in patients older than 50 years.

The presence of calcifications within pulmonary nodules supports the diagnosis of a benign disorder. High-resolution, thin-section CT is the best test for revealing the pattern of calcification. Central, diffuse, laminated, or popcorn patterns of calcification indicate benignity. A stippled pattern or an eccentric calcium deposit does not rule out malignancy. CT densitometry may show occult calcification in nodules that do not have visual evidence of calcium deposits. Nodules with irregular or spiculated margins are most often malignant. Stability of size over a 2-year period is an important sign of benignity. Absence of previous chest radiographs or signs of enlargement of the nodule in a patient over 35 years of age with a history of tobacco use warrants efforts to make a pathologic diagnosis.

Depending on the location and size of the nodule, patients may undergo bronchoscopy with transbronchial biopsy or transthoracic needle aspiration biopsy. When either one or both of these procedures fails to establish a diagnosis, a lung biopsy may be indicated. This recommendation is based on the observation that percutaneous lung aspiration has a sensitivity of 80–90% and a specificity of 95%. Although a relatively accurate test, transthoracic needle aspiration biopsy still does not rule out malignancy with sufficient certainty in a high-risk patient.

It should be recognized, however, that biopsy and aspiration material from patients with suspected tuberculosis can be submitted for mycobacterial culture and result in a high diagnostic yield. More than 95% of patients undergoing bronchoscopy for the diagnosis of sputum negative tuberculosis will have a diagnosis established on the basis of combined histopathologic and microbiologic results. Clinicians must have an appropriately high diagnostic suspicion of tuberculosis, however, to be aware of the diagnosis and know to await cultures before proceeding to lung biopsy.

The approach to lung biopsy has changed dramatically in the past several years with the introduction of video-assisted thoracoscopy for lung biopsy. This procedure can perform a wedge resection of peripheral lung lesions with less morbidity than a full thoracotomy.

The present patient appeared to be at high risk for lung cancer on the basis of the radiographic appearance of the lesion, his age, and the negative histopathologic results of the bronchoscopy and percutaneous needle aspiration. He underwent a lung biopsy that showed granulomas and acid-fast organisms. He was started on isoniazid, rifampin, ethambutol, and pyrazinamide. Cultures from the bronchoscopy specimens (as well as from the biopsy specimen) subsequently grew *M. tuberculosis* sensitive to all drugs.

Clinical Pearls

1. Up to 75% of patients with solitary or multiple pulmonary nodules are asymptomatic, and an equal proportion of these asymptomatic patients have benign versus malignant disease.

2. Overall, 24% of solitary pulmonary nodules in most reported series are due to tuberculosis, with the highest incidence occurring in younger age populations. The proportion of patients with lung cancer is as high as 65% in patients older than 50 years.

3. The likelihood that a lung nodule is malignant relates to the patient's age, the extent of the smoking history, the nodule's diameter, the overall prevalence of malignancy in pulmonary nodules from the patient's region, the radiographic pattern of the edge of the nodule, and the presence of calcification within the nodule.

REFERENCES

1. Toomes H, Delphendahl A, Manke HG, Vogt-Moykopf I. The coin lesion of the lung: a review of 955 resected coin lesions. Cancer 1983;51:534–537.
2. Zwirewich CV, Vedal S, Miller RR, Muller NR. Solitary pulmonary nodule: high-resolution CT and radiologic-pathologic correlation. Radiology 1991;179:469–476.
3. Lillington GA. Management of solitary pulmonary nodules. Dis Mon 1991;37:271–318.
4. Gaeta M, Volta S, Stroscio S, et al. CT "halo sign" in pulmonary tuberculoma. J Comput Assist Tomogr 1992;16:827–828.
5. Jayasundera CI, Attapattu M, Kumarasinghe MP. Atypical presentations of pulmonary tuberculosis diagnosed by fibreoptic bronchoscopy. Postgrad Med J 1993;69:621–623.

PATIENT 17

A 42-year-old man with hemoptysis, a density in the right upper lobe, and a history of tuberculosis

A 42-year-old man presented with a several-month history of cough productive of blood-streaked sputum. The patient denied fever, night sweats, or chills. Four years earlier he had been treated for pulmonary tuberculosis with documented compliance with therapy. The patient also had a history of past intravenous drug abuse and hepatitis.

Physical Examination: Vital signs: normal. General: comfortable. Head: normal. Chest: coarse breath sounds heard over the anterior chest. Heart: normal heart sounds, without murmurs. Abdomen: normal. Neurologic: normal.

Laboratory Findings: Hct 34%, WBC 6400/μl. Electrolytes: normal. Coagulation profile: normal. ABG (room air): pH 7.40, $PaCO_2$ 34 mmHg, PaO_2 91 mmHg. Chest radiograph (shown below): right upper lobe thick-walled cavity with extensive pleural reaction.

Questions: What is the cause of the patient's hemoptysis? What therapy should be undertaken?

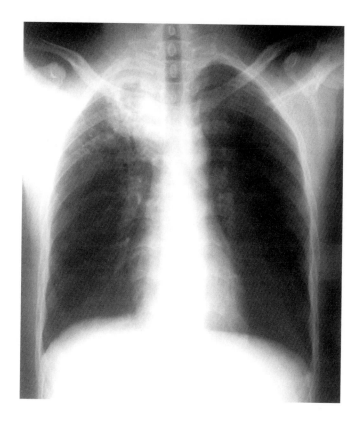

Diagnosis: Aspergilloma (fungus ball) complicating a healed tuberculosis cavity.

Discussion: *Aspergillus* spp. represent a genus of fungi that produce a broad array of clinically distinct pulmonary disorders through disparate pathogenetic mechanisms. Aspergillomas refer to a mass of saprophytic fungal elements that colonize preexisting cavities, frequently producing recurrent hemoptysis. Allergic bronchopulmonary aspergillosis is an immunologically-mediated condition characterized by bronchiectasis, mucus plugging, and wheezing in patients with underlying bronchial asthma. Invasive pulmonary aspergillosis occurs in severely immunocompromised hosts and causes a rapidly progressive and often fatal pulmonary infection. Two additional syndromes, endobronchial pseudomembranous aspergillosis and chronic, necrotizing (semi-invasive) aspergillosis, have been more recently described as unique clinical disorders in patients with varying degrees of immunosuppression.

Of the conditions listed above, aspergillomas are etiologically linked to a history of tuberculosis. Possibly due to regional impairment of airway clearance mechanisms or other ill-defined factors, patients with tuberculous lung cavities develop intracavitary colonization of fungal elements that form masses of entwined hyphae termed "fungus balls." This disorder is not particularly unusual in that one large classic study of 544 patients found that 11% of healed lung cavities of greater than 2.5 cm in diameter had radiographic evidence of fungus balls. After 3 years of additional observation, the percentage of patients with intracavitary fungus balls increased to 17%. Aspergillomas can also complicate cavities that develop from other diseases, such as sarcoidosis or rarely cavitating neoplasms.

The major clinical consequence of aspergilloma is the occurrence of intracavitary hemorrhage and resultant hemoptysis, which can be massive and life-threatening. Nearly all patients with fungus balls will experience at least one episode of airway hemorrhage during their life. The pathogenesis of the hemoptysis in not clearly defined, but may relate to the plethoric formation of hypervascular granulation tissue on the walls of cavities colonized by aspergillomas.

The presence of hemoptysis in a patient with preexisting cavitary disease and characteristic radiographic features suggests the diagnosis of aspergilloma. These radiographic features center on detecting the "crescent sign," which refers to a rim of radiolucent air that surrounds a mass (the aspergilloma) within a cavity. Aspergilloma-containing cavities also have a characteristic feature of being thick-walled with a thickened region of overlying pleura. On CT scans, the fungus ball, which is often attached to the lung on a stalk, may be observed to move within the cavity as the patient changes from the prone to supine position.

Aspergillus spp. can usually be cultured from sputum or bronchoscopy specimens in patients with aspergillomas. Aspergillus serum precipitins are detectable in almost all patients. Neither of these findings, however, is specific for the diagnosis of aspergilloma and may not even indicate the presence of an aspergillus-related disease.

The management of patients with aspergillomas depends on the clinical expression of the disease. Most physicians would simply observe asymptomatic patients when a fungus ball is detected incidentally. Therapeutic interventions should be considered for patients with hemoptysis. Patients with massive, life-threatening hemoptysis should be evaluated for surgical resection of the involved lobe or segment. Surgery is occasionally complicated by difficulties with separating the lung from the thickened pleurae overlying the region of the aspergilloma. Many patients may be poor operative candidates because of limited respiratory reserve due to loss of lung function from the underlying cavitary disease. This limitation is less of a factor in patients with aspergillomas within tuberculous cavities in contrast to patients with sarcoidosis who frequently have more generalized destruction of lung tissue. As an alternative to surgical lung resection, bronchial artery embolization may be attempted, although rebleeding may occur in as many as 20–25% of patients. Patients with nonmassive hemoptysis may be selected for careful observation without invasive interventions because up to 10% of aspergillomas may eventually resolve spontaneously.

Systemic antifungal drug therapy with amphotericin B or ketoconazole has proved ineffective in the management of aspergillomas because drugs do not reach the intracavitary fungal elements. Several small patient series have reported clinical responses when antifungal agents, such as amphotericin B, are directly instilled into the cavity percutaneously or through a bronchoscope channel. Despite the anecdotal nature of these reports, it seems reasonable to instill intracavitary amphotericin for patients with serious degrees of hemoptysis who cannot undergo surgery or bronchial embolization or when patients have failed previous embolization attempts. It is uncertain how amphotericin controls hemoptysis in this condition; the rapidity of the response, however, suggests an intracavitary sclerosing effect rather than benefit from the drug's antifungal properties.

The present patient had the characteristic features of a fungus ball within a preexisting tuberculous cavity. A CT scan confirmed the diagnosis. Because of the small amount of bleeding, the patient was treated with antibiotics for a possible bacterial superinfection. The hemoptysis resolved and the patient remains in outpatient followup without specific intervention directed at the mycetoma.

Clinical Pearls

1. Aspergilloma should be considered in the differential diagnosis of a patient presenting with a history of hemoptysis and previous tuberculosis.

2. Fungus balls can be diagnosed by their characteristic clinical and radiographic features; invasive diagnostic procedures are not necessary unless an underlying cavitating neoplasm is a clinical possibility.

3. Although surgical resection is definitive and usually successful in patients with adequate respiratory reserve, bronchial artery embolization and intracavitary administration of antifungal agents may be alternatives when surgery cannot be performed.

REFERENCES

1. Al-Majed SA, Ashour M, El-Kassimi FA, et al. Management of post-tuberculous complex aspergilloma of the lung: role of surgical resection. Thorax 1990;45:846–849.
2. Massard G, Roeslin N, Wihlm JM, et al. Pleuropulmonary aspergilloma: clinical spectrum and results of surgical treatment. Ann Thorac Surg 1992;54:1159–1164.
3. Gefter WB. The spectrum of pulmonary aspergillosis. J Thorac Imaging 1992;7:56–74.
4. Jackson M, Flower CD, Shneerson JM. Treatment of symptomatic pulmonary aspergilloma with intracavitary instillation of amphotericin B through an indwelling catheter. Thorax 1993;48:928–930.

PATIENT 18

A 43-year-old woman with nausea and vomiting while on antituberculosis therapy

A 43-year-old woman presented with nausea and vomiting of 1 week's duration. A diagnosis of tuberculosis had been made 4 months earlier and she was placed on a regimen of isoniazid, rifampin, pyrazinamide, and ethambutol. The latter two drugs were discontinued 2 months into treatment when culture results indicated that her isolate was pan-sensitive. She denied fever or abdominal pain. There was also a history of alcohol abuse, and the patient admitted to active drinking during the time she was receiving antituberculous therapy.

Physical Examination: Temperature 99.3°F, other vital signs normal. General: thin, uncomfortable appearing woman in obvious discomfort. Head: normal. Neck: shotty cervical adenopathy. Chest: scattered crackles throughout all lung fields. Heart: normal heart sounds, without murmurs. Abdomen: mild right upper quadrant tenderness, without rebound or organomegaly. Extremities: normal. Neurologic: normal.

Laboratory Findings: Hct 26%, WBC 11,400/μl. Serum electrolytes and coagulation profile: normal. Aspartate aminotransferase (SGOT): 482 IU/L, alanine aminotransferase (SGPT): 376 IU/L, total bilirubin: 2.8 mg/dl (1.9 mg/dl direct). Erythrocyte sedimentation rate: 93 mm/hr. Serologic testing for hepatitis B and C: negative.

Questions: What is the likely cause of the patient's nausea and vomiting? How should her antituberculous medications be adjusted, if at all?

Diagnosis: Isoniazid-induced hepatitis.

Discussion: Adverse reactions to antituberculous medications represent a frequent clinical problem that complicates the completion of drug therapy and creates a risk for the development of drug-resistant tuberculosis. Of the drug reactions commonly encountered, hepatotoxicity is often the most puzzling to decipher and difficult to manage.

Hepatotoxicity has been generally stated to occur in 2–10% of patients who are undergoing therapy with regimens that contain isoniazid, pyrazinamide, and rifampin. One recent study, however, indicated that as many as 17% of patients treated with these three drugs for 2 months followed by isoniazid and rifampin for 4 months developed abnormal liver function tests. Most of these patients were aymptomatic and had elevations in transaminase levels less than 5 times normal values. Such patients do not require discontinuation of therapy. As many as 6% of the patients in this study experienced severe rises in transaminase levels. Almost all of these patients were known to be consuming large quantities of alcohol while on antituberculous drug therapy.

Ongoing alcohol consumption is one of the major risk factors for drug-induced liver disease in patients receiving antituberculous medications. These patients should undergo close monitoring of clinical symptoms and liver function tests. Other forms of preexisting liver disease or the coadministration of other potential hepatotoxins can also potentiate liver injury in patients undergoing drug therapy. One study, for instance, identified viral hepatitis as a risk factor for drug-induced disease. This study indicated that 35% of patients who developed symptomatic hepatitis during antituberculous therapy were hepatitis B carriers, as determined by positive surface antigens. Of note, viral carriers had many more severe drug reactions than patients who were noncarriers. Similarly, another group of investigators found evidence of viral hepatitis in 42% of children with symptomatic hepatitis that had been attributed to antituberculous medications.

The mechanism and pattern of liver abnormalities from antituberculosis medications differ from drug to drug. Isoniazid typically causes a rise in transaminases through mechanisms that are not clearly defined. Attempts to link the risk of isoniazid-induced hepatitis to a patient's phenotype status as a rapid or slow acetylator have not yielded uniform results. Testing to determine a patient's acetylation phenotype before initiation of isoniazid therapy is not presently recommended.

Rifampin is also associated with hepatotoxicity, and the combination of isoniazid and rifampin is more hepatotoxic than either given alone. Rifampin also has a more pronounced effect on bilirubin metabolism than isoniazid: it competitively interferes with bilirubin uptake and can cause hyperbilirubinemia without actually damaging the liver. Isolated elevations in bilirubin, therefore, are likely due to rifampin.

Of other commonly used antituberculous drugs, pyrazinamide was frequently reported as a cause of severe hepatitis when it was first introduced, possibly related to the high doses that were at first recommended. At currently employed doses (maximum daily dose is usually 1.5–2.5 gm), hepatitis is rare with pyrazinamide.

Ethambutol is an extremely rare cause of hepatitis, and streptomycin has not been associated with this complication. Of the second-line agents, ethionamide and PAS have been noted to cause hepatitis.

The management of abnormal liver function during multiagent chemotherapy need not be complex. Asymptomatic, mild (less than three times normal) elevations in liver function can be followed in most patients without changing the drug regimen. For symptomatic or larger rises in transaminase levels, it may be necessary to stop all drugs and sequentially reintroduce them, with the agent most likely to cause the abnormality given last. Any drug found to cause a rise in transaminases of more than five times, particularly if associated with symptoms, should be permanently discontinued. While reintroducing drugs, no patient should be left on monotherapy for more than a few days because of the risk of development of drug resistance.

Adjustment of a treatment regimen has major implications for the total duration of therapy. If isoniazid is dropped from the regimen, cure should still be expected using a regimen of rifampin and ethambutol if the organism is pan-sensitive. Although evidence suggests that 6 months of therapy can be adequate in a regimen that does not contain isoniazid, most authorities recommend at least 9 months of treatment. If rifampin is dropped from the regimen, however, an aminoglycoside and one other agent should be added, and treatment continued for at least 18 months.

The present patient's liver enzymes returned to normal after isoniazid was discontinued. Treatment was continued successfully with rifampin and ethambutol for 9 months.

Clinical Pearls

1. Hepatic dysfunction during treatment for active tuberculosis is usually not serious. Mild elevations in the liver function tests in the absence of symptoms do not require alterations in the drug regimen.

2. A careful search for drugs or conditions (alcohol use, viral hepatitis, acetaminophen usage) known to potentiate liver toxicity should be initiated in patients who develop more severe liver dysfunction.

3. Isoniazid is more likely to cause a transaminitis and rifampin a cholestatic picture, although overlap can occur. Patients with symptoms or elevations of liver function tests greater than three times baseline should have all drugs discontinued and readministered one at a time. Drugs associated with a five times or greater rise in transaminases should be permanently discontinued.

REFERENCES

1. Cohn DL, Catlin BJ, Peterson KL, et al. A 62-dose, 6-month therapy for pulmonary and extrapulmonary tuberculosis: a twice weekly, directly observed, and cost-effective regimen. Ann Intern Med 1990;112:407–415.
2. Wu JC, Lee SD, Yeh PF, et al. Isoniazid-rifampin-induced hepatitis in hepatitis B carriers. Gastroenterology 1990;98:502–504.
3. Kumar A, Misra PK, Mehotra R, et al. Hepatotoxicity of rifampin and isoniazid. Is it all drug-induced hepatitis? Am Rev Respir Dis 1991;143:1350–1352.
4. Centers for Disease Control and Prevention. Severe isoniazid-associated hepatitis–New York, 1991–1993. MMWR 1993;42:545–547.

PATIENT 19

A 37-year-old HIV-infected man with a right axillary mass and HIV disease

A 37-year-old man with a 3-year history of HIV infection presented with fever, chills, a nonproductive cough, and right axillary swelling of 3–4 months' duration. He had been treated for syphilis 15 years earlier, and a tuberculin skin test was negative 2 years previously. Medications included zidovudine and ibuprofen.

Physical Examination: Temperature 102°F, other vital signs normal. General: obese, no acute distress. Head: normal. Axilla: tender, firm 2–3 cm lymph node Neck: tender, rubbery right supraclavicular adenopathy. Chest: normal. Heart: normal heart sounds without murmurs. Abdomen: liver span 15 cm by percussion, otherwise normal. Extremities: normal. Neurologic: normal.

Laboratory Findings: Hct 37%, WBC 4,700/μl, Electrolytes: normal. Tuberculin skin test: positive at 11 mm of induration. Erythrocyte sedimentation rate: 115 mm/hr. Chest radiograph: shown below. Sputum smears: negative for acid-fast organisms.

Questions: What is the likely cause of the axillary lymphadenopathy considering the patient's abnormal chest radiograph?

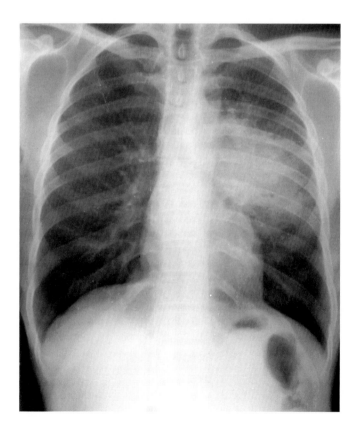

Diagnosis: Tuberculous lymphadenitis.

Discussion: Tuberculous lymphadenitis is one of the more common forms of extrapulmonary tuberculosis and accounts for 20–40% of extrapulmonary disease. It is particularly common in children, and in the adult population it is now a common cause of lymphadenopathy in patients with HIV infection. In the absence of HIV infection, tuberculous lymphadenopathy is usually not associated with systemic symptoms. Patients with HIV infection complicated by tuberculous lymphadenitis often complain of fever and sweats. Pulmonary tuberculosis occurs in only 5–70% of patients with tuberculous lymphadenitis, so a normal chest radiograph does not exclude the diagnosis.

The involved nodes are initially painless but may become tender and occasionally rupture through the skin as the disease progresses. Despite the relative frequency of tuberculous lymphadenitis compared to other forms of extrapulmonary disease, two clinical issues continue to generate controversy and discussion: the proper method of diagnosis and the optimal duration of drug treatment.

For many years it has been said that needle biopsy of tuberculous lymph nodes may produce cutaneous sinus tracts and that excisional biopsy is the preferred diagnostic procedure. However, recent experience indicates that this is not the case. Percutaneous needle biopsy is a safe and effective technique. A large clinical experience has demonstrated that fine-needle aspiration biopsy of peripheral lymph nodes yields a diagnosis in the vast majority of patients, and rarely, if ever, causes sinus tract formation in the antibiotic era. A typical series reviewed 80 patients with proven tuberculous lymphadenitis. A fine-needle aspiration biopsy yielded a diagnosis in 66/80 (83%) of patients. Diagnosis rests on the demonstration of granulomas, acid-fast organisms, or both, with final confirmation determined by positive culture results. Several other series confirm the value of fine (or larger bore, such as a 19-gauge needle) needle aspiration biopsy, making it the diagnostic procedure of choice for evaluation of suspected tuberculous lymphadenitis.

The issue of duration of treatment is still a matter of some debate. Short-course chemotherapy using 6- or 9-month treatment regimens has become the standard approach to patients with pulmonary disease, but this strategy has not been widely accepted for many forms of extrapulmonary tuberculosis to date. However, evidence has been gathering recently that regimens of 6 or 9 months' duration may be associated with excellent cure rates and low relapse rates in tuberculous lymphadenitis. A recent study by the British Thoracic Society of 199 patients with tuberculous lymphadenitis randomized individuals into either 6 or 9 months of treatment and found that a 6-month regimen consisting of 2 months of pyrazinamide, isoniazid, and rifampin, followed by 4 additional months of isoniazid and rifampin alone, was associated with excellent clinical response and a low relapse rate. The results obtained with this regimen were not different from 9-month regimens. Similar results were obtained in a study carried out in children at the Tuberculosis Research Center in Madras. However, an earlier study indicated that a significant (as much as 25%) number of patients may not respond in 6 months' time, so that caution should be used in employing these regimens, and close follow-up is needed.

Several clinical features of the present patient's presentation pointed strongly to the diagnosis of tuberculous lymphadenitis. The history of HIV infection, a newly positive tuberculin skin test, systemic complaints of fever and chills, and the findings of supraclavicular lymph nodes and an abnormal chest radiograph all raised suspicion for a diagnosis of tuberculosis. He had a fine-needle aspiration of the axillary nodes that yielded acid-fast organisms; cultures grew *M. tuberculosis* sensitive to all medications. A sputum culture obtained at the time of admission also grew *M. tuberculosis*. He was treated for 9 months by his physicians (2 months with isoniazid, rifampin, pyrazinamide, and ethambutol followed by 7 months of isoniazid and rifampin) with an excellent clinical response.

Clinical Pearls

1. Tuberculous lymphadenitis is a common form of extrapulmonary tuberculosis. In adults, it occurs most often in patients with HIV infection, who are more likely to have systemic symptoms, such as fever and weight loss, compared to patients with normal immune responses.

2. Fine-needle aspiration biopsy is clearly the initial diagnostic procedure of choice.

3. Short-course chemotherapy may be used to treat tuberculous lymphadenitis, although the clinical response must be carefully monitored.

REFERENCES

1. Behara D, Jindal SK. Short course chemotherapy (9 months) for lymphatic tuberculosis. Indian J Chest Dis Allied Sci 1990;32:73–74.
2. Dandapat MC, Mishra BM, Dash SP, Kar PK. Peripheral lymph node tuberculosis: a review of 80 cases. Br J Surg 1990;77:911–912.
3. Jawahar MS, Sivasubramanian S, Vijayan RK, et al. Short-course chemotherapy for tuberculous lymphadenitis in children. BMJ 1990;301:359–362.
4. Shriner KA, Mathisen GE, Goetz MB. Comparison of mycobacterial lymphadenitis among persons infected with human immunodeficiency virus and seronegative controls. Clin Infect Dis 1992;15:601–605.
5. Campbell IA, Ormerod LP, Friend JA, et al. Six months versus nine months chemotherapy for tuberculosis of lymph nodes: final results. Respir Med 1993;87:621–623.

PATIENT 20

A 38-year-old former quarry worker with a positive tuberculin skin test

A 38-year-old man presented with slowly progressive dyspnea on exertion over the previous 2 years. He had a mild, nonproductive cough but denied fever, night sweats, or weight loss, and had no risk factors for HIV disease. Presently a carpenter, the patient had worked for 2 years as the operator of a quarry rock crusher 10 years earlier. He was unaware of any exposure to tuberculosis.

Physical Examination: Vital signs: normal. General: comfortable. Chest: decreased breath sounds throughout both lungs. Cardiac: normal. Abdomen: normal. Extremities: digital clubbing.

Laboratory Findings: Tuberculin skin test: 10-mm induration. Sputum: negative smears and cultures for acid-fast bacilli. Chest radiograph (below, top): multiple large bullae and a large density in each mid-lung zone. Chest CT (below, bottom): multiple small nodules that coalesce into large densities, one with a central lucency that appears to be a bronchiectatic airway, and many large bullae.

Question: What is the clinical significance of the positive tuberculin skin test?

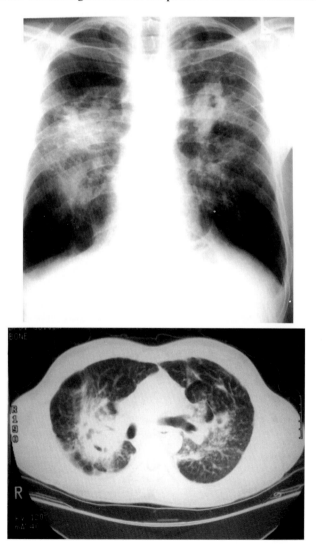

massive fibrosis and tuberculous infection (silicotuberculosis).

e inhalation
of the most
seases that
d in such
, ceramics,
facturing of
lica and the
ng disease.
tion, rubber
are also at
isease. Sili-
of appropri-
th a typical
iffuse small

ry, tubercu-
tially lethal
vent of anti-
of granite
s. Although
on cause of
tuberculosis
ty for work-
cupationally

tuberculosis
the severity
mine work-

unique form of silicosis known as silicoproteinosis after massive exposures to silica dust. These patients appear to be at increased risk for lung infections by *M. kansasii* and *M. avium* as well as *M. tuberculosis*.

The high rate of tuberculosis in workers at risk for silicosis necessitates effective screening programs with tuberculin skin testing in this population. Ideally, skin testing should be integrated with the radiographic screening programs for silicosis in which these workers usually participate. Previously, workers with tuberculin reactions ≥ 10 mm without bacteriologic evidence of active tuberculosis were recommended to receive preventive therapy with isoniazid. Because advanced silicosis shares radiographic features with active tuberculosis, some authorities have argued that these workers should be treated for active tuberculosis if they reacted to tuberculin even when bacteriologic tests were negative.

Current guidelines recommend treatment for patients with silicosis and tuberculin reactions ≥ 10 mm, regardless of age, with the same regimen employed for patients with sputum smear- and culture-negative active tuberculosis. These guidelines call for treatment with at least isoniazid and rifampin for 4 months. Pyrazinamide should be included for the first 2 months. Isoniazid alone for 12 months is an acceptable but less preferable alternative.

Patients with active silicotuberculosis are not candidates for short-course therapy because relapse rates with 6-month regimens are as high as 22%. These patients should be treated with standard multidrug regimens for a minimum of 9 months if they are infected with drug-sensitive organisms.

The present patient had radiographic evidence of multiple parenchymal nodules. These findings combined with a history of silica exposure were sufficient for the diagnosis of silicosis. The positive tuberculin skin test and negative sputum cultures for mycobacteria prompted his physician to initiate multidrug, 4-month regimen in accordance with current guidelines.

ers in South Africa with advanced silicosis, the incidence of tuberculosis is 6%, which is approximately twice the incidence in coworkers with radiographically mild to moderate silicosis. Overall, workers with radiographic evidence of silicosis have about three times the incidence of tuberculosis compared to coworkers without silicosis despite similar degrees and durations of silica exposure. However, even workers exposed to silica who have no radiographic evidence of silicosis have up to a twofold increase in risk for tuberculosis compared with the general population. Interestingly, the risk of developing extrapulmonary tuberculosis is the same as the risk of pulmonary tuberculosis in patients with silicosis. Some patients develop a

Clinical Pearls

1. Workers exposed to silica are at increased risk compared to unexposed workers for developing active tuberculosis after primary infection even in the absence of radiographic evidence of silicosis.

2. Workers with silicosis have a threefold increase in risk for tuberculosis compared to coworkers with comparable dust exposure who do not have silicosis.

3. All patients with silicosis and a tuberculin reaction ≥ 10 mm who are sputum smear- and culture-negative should receive a multidrug regimen for 4 months, regardless of age.

4. Patients with silicosis and active tuberculosis are not candidates for short-course therapy due to unacceptable relapse rates, and must receive a minimum of 9 months of multidrug therapy.

REFERENCES

1. Snider DE. The relationship between tuberculosis and silicosis. Am Rev Respir Dis 1978;118:455–460.
2. Sherson D, Lander F. Morbidity of pulmonary tuberculosis among silicotic and nonsilicotic foundry workers in Denmark. J Occup Med 1990;32:110–113.
3. Hong Kong Chest Service/British Medical Research Council. A controlled clinical comparison of 6 and 8 months of antituberculous chemotherapy in the treatment of patients with silicotuberculosis in Hong Kong. Am Rev Respir Dis 1991;143:262–267.
4. Balaan MR, Banks DE. Silicosis. In Rom WN (ed): Environmental and Occupational Medicine. Boston, Little, Brown, 1992.
5. Cowie, RL. Epidemiology of tuberculosis in gold miners with silicosis. Am J Respir Crit Care Med 1994;150:1460–1462.

PATIENT 21

A 45-year-old man with pulmonary tuberculosis and right hemiparesis

A 45-year-old homeless man undergoing therapy for pulmonary tuberculosis was admitted for the evaluation of right sided motor weakness. He had started therapy with isoniazid, rifampin, pyrazinamide, and ethambutol 10 weeks earlier on the basis of a positive sputum smear for acid-fast bacilli and a chest radiograph appearance of extensive tuberculosis. Sputum cultures had grown *M. tuberculosis,* but drug susceptibility tests were still pending. The patient had been compliant with therapy, and sputum smears converted to negative after 8 weeks of therapy. He had been gaining strength, although he walked with difficulty because of severe cachexia and generalized weakness related to his chronic alcoholism. During the last several days, his walking became progressively more difficult and it was noticed that his right leg was weak.

Physical Examination: Vital signs: normal. General: mildly confused, oriented to person and place, cachectic. Head: poor dentition, atraumatic. Lungs: markedly decreased breath sounds on left. Abdomen: no hepatosplenomegaly or ascites. Neurologic: cranial nerves intact, motor 3/5 on right, 4/5 on left, sensory intact.

Laboratory Findings: WBC 8,900/μl, Hct 38%. Electrolytes, renal indices, liver function tests: normal. Sputum: smear for acid-fast bacilli negative. CSF: protein 51 mg/dl, glucose 62 mg/dl, cells: WBC 0/μl, RBC 122/ml. Chest radiograph: shown below left. CT of head: shown below right.

Questions: What is the most likely cause of this patient's brain lesion? How should it be managed?

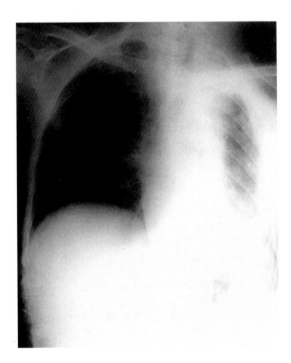
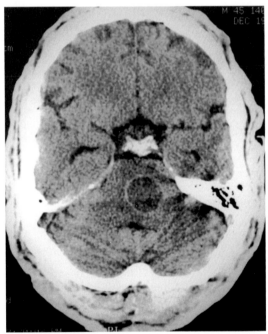

Diagnosis: Intracranial tuberculoma in a patient with pulmonary tuberculosis.

Discussion: Tuberculosis of the central nervous system (CNS) accounts for nearly 10% of cases of extrapulmonary disease in the United States. Children are especially prone to develop this form of tuberculosis. Autopsy studies indicate that the majority of children who die with tuberculosis have pathologic evidence of CNS infection.

Tuberculous meningitis is a manifestation of an inflammatory response to the antigenic stimulation that occurs when a tubercle in the brain parenchyma ruptures and spills organisms into the meningeal space. In contrast, tuberculomas occur when the tubercle in the brain becomes encased in a fibrous capsule, effectively walling off the antigenic tuberculoprotein from the inflammatory cells of the host. As the tuberculoma enlarges, symptoms develop of a space-occupying mass lesion rather than an inflammatory process. Some patients, however, may have the coexistence of tuberculomas with tuberculous meningitis. Most tuberculomas occur singly, although some patients have multiple tuberculomas in different regions of the brain. Approximately one-fourth of patients with tuberculomas have accompanying radiographic evidence of pulmonary tuberculosis. Rare patients may develop symptomatic tuberculomas arising "paradoxically" during the course of appropriate drug therapy for pulmonary tuberculosis. These lesions may resolve with continued treatment.

Seizures are the most common, and often the only, manifestations of tuberculomas. Focal neurologic findings are related to the area of brain involved, although some patients will manifest only symptoms of elevated intracranial pressure. Lumbar puncture is not helpful in the diagnosis, as findings are usually normal in the absence of concomitant meningitis, reflecting the prevention of communication between the tuberculoma and the subarachnoid space by the capsule.

The appearance of tuberculomas on head CT scans is characteristic, with features of an avascular mass that enhances in either a uniform or ring-like pattern, usually with surrounding edema. MRI scans may be more sensitive than CT in detecting small tuberculomas. Radiographic findings are not sufficiently specific, however, to confirm the diagnosis, which requires tissue biopsy or needle aspiration.

Drug therapy for tuberculomas is the same as for pulmonary tuberculosis, although duration of treatment should be 9–12 months. Some tuberculosis experts advocate treating patients with tuberculomas for 18–24 months. Steroids may benefit patients who have evidence of elevated intracranial pressure. Surgery is generally not indicated, because recovery is better in patients who receive medical therapy alone compared to patients who undergo surgical resection of their lesions. The exception relates to rare patients whose tuberculomas undergo caseous liquefaction, producing a tuberculous brain abscess that usually requires surgical excision in addition to antituberculous chemotherapy.

The present patient had a chest radiograph that was compatible with the diagnosis of pulmonary tuberculosis and a head CT scan that demonstrated a ring-enhancing lesion. A needle aspiration of the brain lesion was consistent with granulomatous inflammation. Smears and cultures of the aspirate were negative for acid-fast bacilli. The neurologic symptoms slowly resolved after 8 weeks of continued antituberculous therapy. The patient completed 12 months of therapy without further neurologic complications.

Clinical Pearls

1. Tuberculomas produce symptoms due to a mass effect on the brain, leading to seizures and focal neurologic findings.

2. Lumber puncture findings are usually normal when tuberculomas are present in the absence of meningitis.

3. Tuberculomas may arise while the patient is receiving appropriate antituberculous chemotherapy for another focus of disease; this does not represent a treatment failure.

4. CT and MRI findings of a contrast-enhanced avascular lesion that may be single or multiple are characteristic for tuberculomas. Definitive diagnosis depends on biopsy or needle aspiration demonstrating necrotizing granulomas.

5. Medical therapy with standard antituberculous medications alone leads to a better outcome than when combined with surgical resection of tuberculomas, except in the rare occasions when the tuberculoma liquefies to produce a tuberculous brain abscess.

REFERENCES

1. Harder E, Al-Kawi MZ, Carney P. Intracranial tuberculoma: conservative management. Am J Med 1983;74:570–576.
2. Bahemuka M, Murungi JH. Tuberculosis of the nervous system: a clinical, radiological, and pathological study of 39 consecutive cases in Riyadh, Saudi Arabia. J Neurol Sci 1989;90:67–76.
3. Humphries M. The management of tuberculous meningitis. Thorax 1992;47:577–581.
4. White AE, Davies KG, Anwar S, et al. Cerebral tuberculoma. Br J Clin Pract 1994;48:222–223.
5. Selvapandian S, Rajshekar V, Chandy Mj, Idikula J. Predictive value of computed tomography-based diagnosis of intracranial tuberculoma. Neurosurgery 1994;35:845–850.
6. Konsuoglu SS, Ozcan C, Ozmenoglu M, et al. Intracranial tuberculoma: clinical and computerized tomographic findings. Israel J Med Sci 1994;30:153–157.

PATIENT 22

A 36-year-old man with pulmonary tuberculosis and lung masses

A 36-year-old man was referred to the hospital because of a positive sputum culture for *Mycobacterium tuberculosis* and an abnormal chest radiograph. The patient had been evaluated 6 weeks earlier at an outside clinic for fever. Sputum acid-fast smears were negative, and mycobacterial cultures had been sent to an outside laboratory. The patient had a history of alcohol and tobacco use. He had otherwise been healthy.

Physical Examination: Temperature 99.6°F. General: ill-appearing. Chest: crackles at the right apex. The remainder of the examination was normal.

Laboratory Findings: Hct 36%, WBC 5,600/μl, platelets normal. Electrolytes and liver function tests: normal. Chest radiograph (below): density in the right apex of the lung, cavitary lesion in the left lower lung field. Sputum culture results: *M. tuberculosis* sensitive to all tested drugs except isoniazid.

Question: Are there any diagnostic concerns other than the presence of active pulmonary tuberculosis?

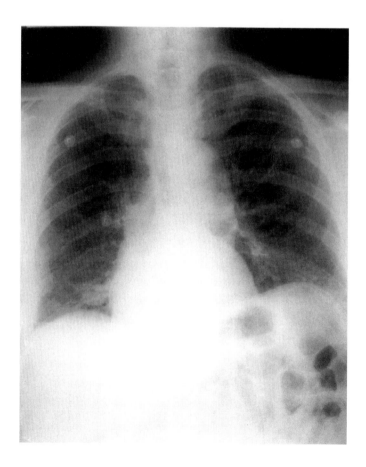

Diagnosis: Bilateral non-small-cell carcinoma in a patient with active pulmonary tuberculosis.

Discussion: An intriguing association between pulmonary tuberculosis and lung cancer exists that can present the unwary clinician with diagnostic hazards. Both conditions can present with a progressive illness characterized by pulmonary symptoms and generalized debility. Also, the chest radiograph in these two conditions can have overlapping features. For instance, tuberculosis may produce tuberculomas or other mass-like lesions than can simulate a lung tumor. Similarly, some lung cancers—most notably squamous cell—may cavitate, giving the radiographic appearance of cavitary tuberculosis.

An association may also exist in the pathogenesis of these two disorders. It has been long considered that patients with malignancy have a higher incidence of developing active tuberculosis, although supporting evidence is not entirely clear. Recent patient series indicate that patients with lung cancer who have positive tuberculin skin tests have a relatively high rate of developing active tuberculosis. It appears, however, that this reactivation rate relates more to the use of chemotherapeutic agents and corticosteroids than to the underlying cancer. Because of the limited survival of most patients with lung cancer, it is unclear whether these patients who have a positive tuberculin test should be treated with isoniazid prophylaxis.

It has also been long suspected that a history of tuberculosis may increase the risk of lung cancer. Up to 25% of patients dying of bronchogenic carcinoma have autopsy evidence of healed or active tuberculous lesions. This compares with a 7% incidence of tuberculous lesions in patients dying of other disorders. Similarly, an epidemiologic study from China of 1405 patients with lung cancer and 1495 control subjects determined that patients with a history of tuberculosis had a 50% increase in the incidence of lung cancer after controlling for the effects of smoking.

Although the association is not entirely accepted, if tuberculosis does promote lung cancer, pathogenic mechanisms are unclear, especially considering that many of the malignancies occur away from the site of tuberculous infection or in the contralateral lung. The so-called scar carcinoma has long been believed to be a hallmark of the relationship between prior tuberculous inflammation leading to a scar that then proceeds to malignant degeneration. Some have suggested, however, that the "scar" found adjacent to some lung cancers is actually a secondary desmoplastic reaction initiated by the malignancy.

In the present patient, the two discrete masses noted on the chest radiograph suggested the presence of a pulmonary malignancy. The patient underwent fiberoptic bronchoscopy and transbronchial biopsy of the right upper lobe and left lower lobe lesions on two separate occasions. Both masses proved to be non-small-cell cancers, most likely squamous cell carcinomas. The patient was initiated on antituberculous therapy for the positive sputum culture for *M. tuberculosis* and is awaiting a staging evaluation.

Clinical Pearls

1. Tuberculosis and lung cancer may mimic each other radiographically. Patients with tuberculosis and radiographs with mass-like lesions that do not improve after appropriate chemotherapy should raise the suspicion of malignancy.

2. Recent series demonstrate an increased incidence of tuberculosis among patients with lung cancer, which may relate to the use of immunosuppressive agents in patients with advanced malignancies.

3. Patients with a history of tuberculosis appear to be at increased risk for bronchogenic carcinoma, independent of other risk factors.

4. Although radiographic screening for lung cancer is not recommended for any patient population, physicians should maintain a high level of suspicion for lung cancer when following patients after completion of tuberculosis chemotherapy.

REFERENCES
1. Zheng W, Blot WJ, Liao ML, et al. Lung cancer and prior tuberculosis infection in Shanghai. Br J Cancer 1987;56:501–504.
2. Alhashimi MM, Citron ML, Fossieck BE, et al. Lung cancer, tuberculin reactivity, and isoniazid. South Med J 1988;81:337–340.
3. Dacosta NA, Kinare SG. Association of lung carcinoma and tuberculosis. J Postgrad Med 1991;37:185–189.
4. Nagata N, Nikaido Y, Kido M, et al. Terminal pulmonary infections in patients with lung cancer. Chest 1993;103:1739–1742.

PATIENT 23

A 46-year-old man with drug-resistant tuberculosis

A 46-year-old man returned for evaluation because of a positive sputum culture for drug-resistant *M. tuberculosis*. Four months earlier, he had been diagnosed with pulmonary tuberculosis on the basis of positive sputum smears and treated with isoniazid, rifampin, pyrazinamide, and ethambutol. Sensitivity results from sputum now revealed that the organism was resistant to both isoniazid and rifampin. The patient had never taken antituberculous medications before the onset of his present illness. He had a history of alcohol abuse but was HIV-negative. He had no known contact with anyone with drug-resistant tuberculosis.

Physical Examination: Temperature 101.2°F, other vital signs normal. General: thin-appearing, no acute distress. Head: normal. Chest: few crackles at the right apex. Heart: normal heart sounds. Abdomen: normal.

Laboratory Findings: Hct 42%, WBC 8200/µl, electrolytes: normal. HIV-antibody test: negative. Chest radiograph: right apical fibronodular infiltrate.

Questions: What is the nature of this patient's drug resistance? What antibiotic regimen should be instituted?

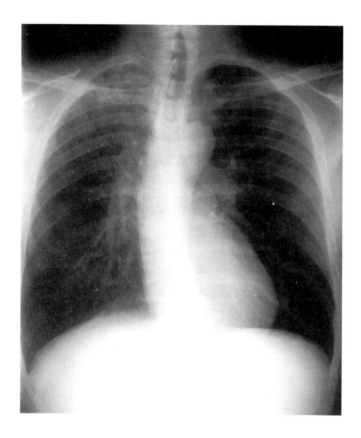

Diagnosis: Primary drug-resistant tuberculosis in a patient without HIV infection.

Discussion: Drug resistance in tuberculosis is classified as primary or secondary, depending on the history of previous antituberculous therapy. Primary resistance occurs in patients who have never taken antituberculous drugs. Secondary resistance develops as a consequence of inadequate drug regimens typically characterized by erratic administration or incorrect drug selection.

Soon after the introduction of streptomycin in the 1940s, two striking observations were made. First, patients demonstrated rapid and dramatic improvement in symptoms, chest x-rays, and culture results after the initiation of streptomycin. Second, initial improvement was followed in a large percentage of patients by relapses caused by resistant organisms. Soon thereafter, experimental evidence revealed that in any population of mycobacteria, the proportion of naturally occurring organisms that were resistant to any one of the first-line antibacterial agents was between 1 in 10^6 and 1 in 10^8. Therefore, the chance that an organism is primarily resistant to two of the first-line drugs would be on the order of 1 in 10^{14} (i.e., $10^6 \times 10^8$). These observations have led to the principle of multidrug therapy for all patients with active tuberculosis, and the corollary principle that a physician should *never* add a single drug to an antituberculous regimen that is failing.

In recognition of these principles, the most recent recommendations of the American Thoracic Society and the Centers for Disease Control state that in a region where the frequency of resistance to isoniazid is known to be >4%, four-drug initial therapy should be instituted in all newly diagnosed cases of tuberculous, pending availability of culture results.

Multidrug resistance (defined as resistance to two or more of the first-line anti-tuberculous agents) is associated with substantially increased morbidity and mortality as compared with disease due to pansensitive organisms. Of all the first-line agents, rifampin is clearly the best available, and studies from the British Medical Research Council in the 1970s and 1980s indicate that if rifampin cannot be used, prolonged treatment regimens of at least 18 months with other agents are necessary. More recent data indicate that even in the most experienced hands, tuberculosis resistant to at least isoniazid and rifampin has a mortality of nearly 40%.

Because sensitivity testing from the patient in this case revealed disease resistant to both isoniazid and rifampin, an aminoglycoside (streptomycin) and a quinolone (ciprofloxacin) were combined with ethambutol and pyrazinamide as a four-drug regimen. Aminoglycosides are bactericidal with excellent *in vitro* activity against *M. tuberculosis*. Quinolones are second-line drugs that have bacteriostatic but good *in vitro* activity against *M. tuberculosis* but are better tolerated than other second-line agents. In the case of tuberculosis resistant to rifampin, treatment most be prolonged and closely monitored to ensure that all drugs are taken as prescribed to prevent both adverse effects and the development of even more resistant isolates. The present patient's sputum cultures became sterile, and he improved with an apparent cure of his tuberculosis.

Clinical Pearls

1. A high rate of secondary drug resistance in a population indicates ongoing problems with tuberculosis control efforts. A high rate of primary resistance may indicate problems with tuberculosis control in the past or possibly rapid spread of the disease through a vulnerable population.

2. Initial regimens for the treatment of tuberculosis should always contain two or more drugs, and in regions where there is a high rate of drug resistance (>4%), as many as four drugs should constitute initial empirical therapy.

3. NEVER add a single drug to a failing regimen for tuberculosis. At least two drugs to which the organism is susceptible should be added simultaneously.

REFERENCES

1. David HL. Probability distribution of drug-resistant mutants in unselected populations of *Mycobacterium tuberculosis*. Appl Microbiol 1970;20:810–814.
2. Goble M, Iseman MD, Madsen L, et al. Treatment of 171 patients with pulmonary tuberculosis resistant to isonaizid and rifampin. N Engl J Med 1993;328:527–532.
3. American Thoracic Society. Treatment of tuberculosis and tuberculosis infection in adults and children. Am J Respir Crit Care Med 1994;149:1359–1375.

PATIENT 24

A 37-year-old man with multidrug-resistant tuberculosis and poor compliance with therapy

A 37-year-old man presented complaining of fever, cough, and weight loss. The patient had a history of tuberculosis diagnosed 2½ years earlier, and the initial isolates were sensitive to all drugs. He was treated at that time with isoniazid, rifampin, and pyrazinamide, which he took sporadically. Over the ensuing 2½ years, he attended clinic irregularly and sputum cultures remained positive for *M. tuberculosis*. Most recent isolates were resistant to isoniazid and rifampin. The patient had never received more than 3 weeks of uninterrupted antituberculosis therapy.

Physical Examination: Temperature 99°F, remainder of vital signs normal. General: chronically ill-appearing man. Head: normal. Chest: scattered crackles throughout all lung fields. Heart: normal heart sounds without murmurs. Abdomen: normal. Neurologic: normal.

Laboratory Findings: Hct 45%, WBC 4,700/μl. Electrolytes: normal. Liver function tests: normal. HIV antibody: negative. Chest radiograph: bilateral upper lung zone fibronodular infiltrates.

Question: What should be done to assure proper therapy for this patient with multidrug-resistant tuberculosis?

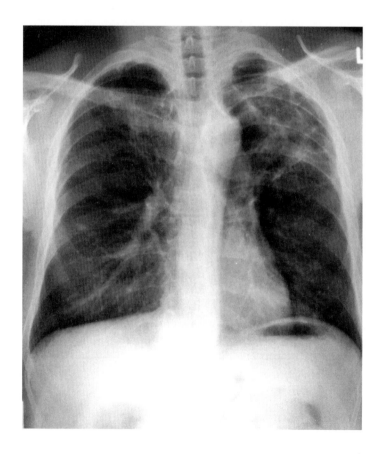

Diagnosis: Noncompliance with antituberculosis medication leading to the development of secondary multidrug-resistant tuberculosis.

Discussion: Numerous studies indicate that only about one-half of patients on a given medical regimen will adhere to it, regardless of the illness for which the drugs were prescribed. For patients with tuberculosis in urban areas, compliance may be far lower. In a landmark report, follow-up data were obtained on nearly 300 consecutive patients discharged from a New York City hospital with a diagnosis of active tuberculosis. Only 11% of patients adhered to the antituberculosis regimen that had been prescribed for self-administration.

The consequences of erratic or incomplete self-administration of drugs are several. First, the patient with tuberculosis will have little chance of a cure. Second, the patient will remain infectious and spread disease to other vulnerable individuals. Third, and perhaps most significant, erratic administration of medication leads to the development of drug-resistant tuberculosis, as occurred in the present patient. This last consequence is of enormous import because the likelihood of cure drops dramatically for patients with multidrug-resistant tuberculosis.

Unfortunately, it is difficult to predict with a high degree of certainty which patients will be noncompliant with therapy. Noncompliance with antituberculosis therapy has been recognized from the earliest days of the antibiotic era, and it may be more common than with other illnesses for two reasons. First, side effects from antituberculous medications are fairly common, and second, patients on antituberculous therapy often experience a rapid improvement in symptoms and may fail to recognize the importance of continuing to take medication when they are feeling well. Therefore, experienced public health officials and clinicians have urged the widespread institution of programs of directly observed therapy (DOT) for the treatment of patients with tuberculosis. DOT programs typically have the patient come to a clinic on an outpatient basis to receive medication while observed by a nurse or other provider. Incentives, such as food or cash, are often provided to increase attendance. Results of such programs have been quite positive in the past. A recent large study from Texas indicated that a DOT program was associated with a decrease in the rate of multidrug-resistance as well as the relapse rate for all cases seen in their clinic over a nearly 10-year period.

DOT programs are now widely available in the United States and are usually administered through the local department of health, although some hospital-based programs are available. Using this approach, at least 90% of patients can be treated to completion of therapy in a humane and compassionate manner. However, despite all efforts, there will remain a few recalcitrant patients for whom coercive measures, such as long-term detention, may be in order. At present 39 states have power to issue detention orders. Physicians caring for patients with a history of noncompliance or who are believed to be at risk for noncompliance should work closely with their local health department to monitor the course of treatment. The burden is on the treating physician to assure treatment to completion, given the public health threat posed by tuberculosis.

The present patient was entered into a DOT program and completed a course of multidrug therapy that resulted in a cure of his tuberculosis.

Clinical Pearls

1. Compliance with antituberculosis therapy in an individual patient is difficult to predict, and noncompliance represents a major public health hazard. The burden is on the treating clinician to ensure compliance.

2. Programs of directly observed therapy (DOT) can improve compliance and are associated with a lower frequency of secondary drug resistance and relapse.

3. For patients who do not comply with DOT, more coercive detention programs may be indicated because of the threat to the public health.

REFERENCES
1. Brudney K, and Dobkin J. Resurgent tuberculosis in New York City: human immunodeficiency virus, homelessness, and the decline of tuberculosis control programs. Am Rev Respir Dis 1991;144:745–749.
2. Gostin LO. Controlling the resurgent tuberculosis epidemic: a 50-state survey of TB statutes and proposals for reform. JAMA 1993;269:255–261.
3. Sumartojo E. When tuberculosis treatment fails: a social behavorial account of patient adherence. Am Rev Respir Dis 1993;147:1311–1320.
4. Weis SE, Slocum PC, Blais FX, et al. The effect of directly observed therapy on the rates of drug resistance and relapse in tuberculosis. N Engl J Med 1994;330:1179–1184.

PATIENT 25

A 31-year-old man with HIV infection, fever, and mediastinal lymphadenopathy

A 31-year-old man, known to be seropositive for HIV, presented with fever. He had a past history of Pneumocystis pneumonia. The patient denied respiratory or other systemic complaints.

Physical Examination: Temperature 102.3°F, other vital signs normal. General: thin, comfortable. Lymph nodes: normal. The remainder of the examination was unremarkable.

Laboratory Findings: CBC, electrolytes, liver function tests, and coagulation profile: normal. CD4+ cell count: 115/μl. Chest radiograph: bilateral hilar and mediastinal lymphadenopathy. Chest CT: mediastinal lymphadenopathy with central necrosis. Gallium[67] scan: uptake in the mediastinal and left hilar lymph nodes. Transbronchial needle aspiration with a core biopsy specimen of mediastinal lymph nodes: granuloma with rare acid-fast organisms. Aspirate cultures: *Mycobacterium avium-intracellulare.*

Question: Should the patient be treated for lymphadenitis due to *M. avium-intracellulare?*

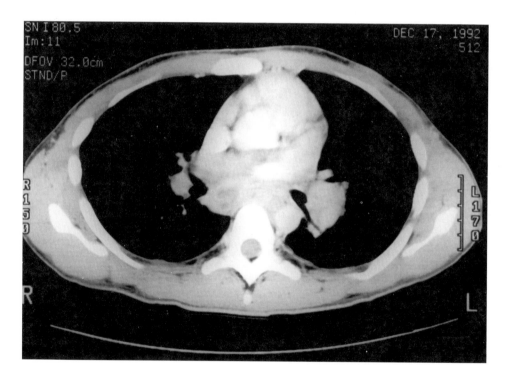

Diagnosis: Mediastinal lymphadenitis due to *Mycobacterium avium-intracellulare*.

Discussion: Lymphadenitis due to *M. tuberculosis* is the most common extrapulmonary form of tuberculosis in most series of non–HIV-infected patients. In patients with AIDS, tuberculous lymphadenitis is also common, and intrathoracic adenopathy as a manifestation of tuberculosis in this population is a well-recognized presentation of disease. In contrast, although lymphadenitis caused by nontuberculous mycobacteria has been noted in children, it is rare in adults.

In adults, infections due to *M. avium* complex, although associated with true pathology in the occasional immunocompetent patient, have been recognized as an important cause of morbidity and mortality in immunocompromised patients, particularly those infected with HIV. In the HIV population, disease due to *M. avium* is generally a disseminated infection that presents with systemic symptoms.

In children with lymphadenitis due to nontuberculous mycobacteria, the disease is difficult, if not impossible, to distinguish clinically or even pathologically from tuberculous lymphadenitis. All 86 children with nontuberculous mycobacterial lymphadenitis in one series had granulomatous inflammation on biopsy, with a substantial number having acid-fast organisms on histopathologic examination. Most of the children were less than 5 years of age, and the disease invariably was confined to the face and neck (although CT scans of the chest were not part of the routine evaluation). All children were treated surgically, with recurrence noted in 6%. In a smaller series, more than twice as many cases of nontuberculous compared with tuberculous lymphadenitis was found in a population of children less than 15 years of age, and the diseases could be distinguished only by culture of the lymph nodes.

The most recent large series comparing tuberculous and nontuberculous lymphadenitis was published by a group from western Australia. In 172 patients with culture-proven mycobacterial lymphadenitis, the distribution of causative organisms differed radically with age. In 118 cases in children under 7, the disease was caused by *M. tuberculosis* in 4%, *M. avium* complex in 74%, and *M. scrofulaceum* in 20%. In contrast, among 54 cases occurring in adults, the causative organisms were *M. tuberculosis* in 89%, *M. avium* complex in 2%, and *M. scrofulaceum* in 4%. Patients with disease due to *M. tuberculosis* were more likely to have a longer duration of symptoms before diagnosis and more local complications. Disease confined to the head and neck was more likely to be due to nontuberculous mycobacteria. Patients with tuberculosis responded well to medical therapy, whereas patients with nontuberculous disease were generally treated with surgery, with recurrence in 10%.

Although in the past nontuberculous lymphadenitis was treated as a surgical disease, recent improvements in drug therapy have made medical therapy a realistic option. Regimens consisting of rifampin (or rifabutin), ethambutol, and clarithromycin have been effective in the treatment of infections due to *M. avium* complex in normal hosts. However, there are few data on the treatment of this condition in immunocompromised patients.

In the present patient, a positive culture for *M. avium* complex is obvious evidence of disease in a patient with AIDS. Mediastinal adenopathy represents an unusual manifestation of *M. avium* disease, and this patient's presentation stresses the importance of making a definitive diagnosis in patients with unexplained adenopathy. The patient was started on a regimen of clarithromycin (500 mg b.i.d.), rifampin, and ethambutol, with some initial improvement in fever. However, 9 months after presentation, the patient developed disseminated infection with *M. avium* and died.

Clinical Pearls

1. Nontuberculous mycobacteria, when cultured from lymph nodes of symptomatic patients with granulomatous adenitis, should be considered as a pathogen.

2. Lymphadenitis due to nontuberculous mycobacteria is most commonly a disease of children but in patients with HIV infection may be a manifestation of disseminated infection with *M. avium* complex.

3. Surgical therapy for nontuberculous lymphadenitis had been standard therapy; however, currently a trial of drug therapy may be warranted in appropriate cases with the agents that have recently shown substantial activity against these organisms.

REFERENCES

1. Joshi W, Davidson PM, Jones PG, et al. Non-tuberculous mycobacterial lymphadenitis in children. Eur J Pediatr 1989;148:751–754.
2. Pang SC. Mycobacterial lymphadenitis in western Australia. Tuber Lung Dis 1992;73:362–367.
3. Colville A. Retrospective review of culture-positive mycobacterial lymphadenitis cases in children in Nottingham, 1979–1990. Eur J Clin Microbiol Infect Dis 1993;12:192–195.

PATIENT 26

A 42-year-old man with asthma and a positive tuberculin skin test

A 42-year-old man presented to the hospital with an asthma exacerbation. The patient was a bakery worker with a long history of asthma that had required intubation and mechanical ventilation on at least two occasions in the past. He averaged three to four hospitalizations per year for the past 3 years, during which he often required systemic steroid therapy. Medications on admission included an inhaled beta-agonist and inhaled steroids. A tuberculin test done 1 month before admission was positive at 16 mm. He denied fever, chills, weight loss, or a cough.

Physical Examination: Respiratory rate: 22, other vital signs normal. General: well-developed man in mild respiratory distress. Head: normal. Chest: expiratory wheezes. Heart: normal heart sounds with no murmurs or rub. Abdomen: normal.

Laboratory Findings: CBC and electrolytes: normal. Peak flow rate: 180 L/min. ABG (room air): pH 7.43, PCO_2 33 mmHg, PO_2 63 mmHg. Chest radiograph: shown below. Liver function tests: normal. HIV antibody: negative.

Question: How should the patient be managed for his positive tuberculin skin test?

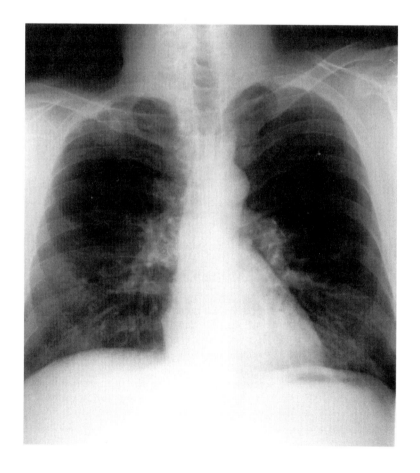

Diagnosis: Asymptomatic tuberculous infection in a patient with difficult-to-control asthma.

Discussion: The presence of a positive PPD skin test in a patient who may require systemic corticosteroid therapy should prompt a consideration of isoniazid preventive therapy. The decision to initiate preventive therapy depends on an analysis in an individual patient of the relative risks of reactivation of the underlying tuberculosis infection and the risks of promoting isoniazid-induced adverse reactions.

The lifetime risk of developing active tuberculosis in general patient populations who have a positive PPD skin test is estimated to be 5–10%. This risk may markedly increase, however, in the presence of comorbid disease. Silicosis, for instance, is well-documented to increase the risk for reactivation tuberculosis. As many as one-third of patients with silicosis and a positive PPD skin test will develop active tuberculosis within 5 years of the initial infection unless treated with preventive therapy. Patients with HIV infection have the highest rate of developing active tuberculosis (10% *per year*) compared to any other patient group. At the other extreme, patients with diabetes have only twice the risk of reactivating a tuberculous infection compared to patients without underlying disease. Conditions with intermediate risks for active tuberculosis include malnutrition, malignancy, and the administration of immunosuppressive agents.

In considering the risk for active tuberculosis in patients with postive PPD skin tests and asthma that is intermittently corticosteroid dependent, physicians should recognize that asthma itself does not increase this risk. Corticosteroids, however, can depress cellular immunity and promote reactivation disease. The American Thoracic Society recommends isoniazid preventive therapy for PPD positive patients who require corticosteroid doses equivalent to >15 mg of prednisone a day for longer than 2–3 weeks. Although based on incomplete data, the preponderance of clinical investigations support this recommendation.

A case controlled study in asthmatic South African gold miners demonstrated no increased risks of active disease when patients were treated with 10–40 mg of prednisone on an alternate-day regimen. One additional study did not note an increased rate of active tuberculosis development when patients were treated with 10–15 mg of prednisone daily.

Any patient with a positive PPD skin test regardless of the dose of corticosteroids used should be evaluated for the presence of active tuberculosis with a chest radiograph. If the radiograph does not show evidence of active disease, the dose and duration of planned corticosteroid therapy can determine the need for preventive therapy.

The present patient was treated with bronchodilators and intravenous corticosteroids and rapidly responded to therapy. His chest radiograph demonstrated a calcified right upper nodule that had been stable for several years. Sputum cultures for mycobacterium had been previously been evaluated and found to be negative. The patient was discharged on a regimen of inhaled bronchodilators and 40 mg of prednisone daily with a plan to discontinue the prednisone within 2–3 weeks. Because of the short duration anticipated for the corticosteroid therapy, the patient was not treated with isoniazid therapy.

Clinical Pearls

1. Patients with positive tuberculin tests who require steroid therapy for another disorder should be carefully evaluated for evidence of active tuberculosis.

2. Patients with positive tuberculin tests on fairly high doses of prednisone (> 15 mg/day or the equivalent) may be candidates for isoniazid preventive therapy, although the risk of developing active tuberculosis is difficult to quantify.

3. Patients with positive tuberculin tests treated with corticosteroids in whom isoniazid preventive therapy is deferred should be monitored closely during therapy for signs and symptoms of active tuberculosis.

REFERENCES

1. Cowie RL, King LM. Pulmonary tuberculosis in corticosteroid-treated asthmatics. S Afr Med J 1987;72:849–850.
2. Bateman ED, Wolmarans KW, White NW, Ainslie GM. Corticosteroid treatment and the risk of active tuberculosis in patients with chronic interstitial lung disease. Am Rev Respir Dis 1991;143:A54.
3. Shaikh WA. Pulmonary tuberculosis in patients treated with inhaled beclomethasone. Allergy 1992;47(4 part 1): 327–330.
4. Bateman ED. Is tuberculosis chemoprophylaxis necessary for patients receiving corticosteroids for respiratory disease? Respir Med 1993;87:485–487.

PATIENT 27

A 28-year-old man with HIV infection and right-sided chest pain

A 28-year-old man with known HIV infection presented with fever and vague right-sided chest discomfort of 2–3 weeks' duration. The patient denied cough, sputum production, or history of tuberculosis exposure. He had never undergone tuberculin skin testing or experienced an opportunistic infection. He did have an episode of bacterial pneumonia 7 months before admission and a distant history of treated syphilis.

Physical Examination: Temperature 99°F, other vital signs normal. General: comfortable. Head: normal. Chest: diminished breath sounds at the right base, with dullness to percussion. Heart: normal heart sounds, without murmurs. Abdomen: normal. Neurologic: normal.

Laboratory Findings: Hct 40%, WBC 7,400/μl. Electrolytes, liver function tests, coagulation profile: normal. Chest radiograph (shown below): right pleural effusion without apparent parenchymal abnormality. Pleural fluid analysis: straw-colored fluid, pH 7.38, protein 4.0 g/L, white blood cell count 1875/μl, (60% lymphocytes).

Questions: What is the likely cause of the effusion? What should be the approach to diagnosis and treatment?

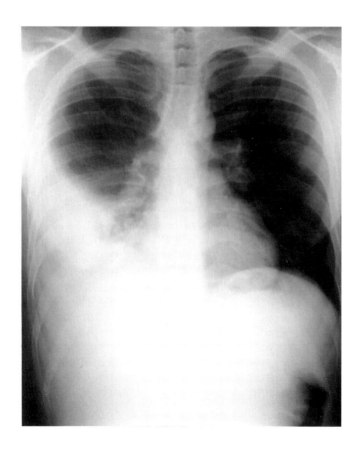

Diagnosis: Tuberculous pleurisy.

Discussion: The finding of a unilateral, lymphocyte-predominant, exudative pleural effusion in a young, previously healthy patient strongly suggests a diagnosis of tuberculous pleurisy. The presence of HIV infection greatly extends the differential diagnosis, however, to pathogens and clinical disorders that typically do not affect the pleurae in immunocompetent hosts. As a result, the diagnostic approach to patients with AIDS and a pleural effusion requires consideration of a more extensive differential diagnosis.

A retrospective review of 222 consecutive hospitalized patients with AIDS determined that 27% of patients had a pleural effusion at some time during their hospitalization. In 66% of patients, the cause was determined to be infectious, with the leading pathogens being bacterial (with parapneumonic effusion) in 18 patients, *Pneumocystis carinii* in 9, *Mycobacterium tuberculosis* in 5, septic emboli in 2, *Nocardia asteroides* in 2, *Cryptococcus neoformans* in 2, and *Mycobacterium avium* in 1. Of the noninfectious etiologies, hypoalbuminemia and heart failure accounted for the majority of pleural effusions, with Kaposi's sarcoma responsible for only one case. Of note, large effusions were more likely to be caused by tuberculosis or Kaposi's sarcoma. Multiple case reports identify lymphoma and histoplasmosis as additional causes of pleural effusions in patients with AIDS.

Pleural effusions due to Kaposi's sarcoma have characteristic features of a serosanguinous appearance, with a mononuclear cell predominance. All patients have a high pleural fluid protein within the exudative range. Occasional patients have been reported with chylothoraces most probably from obstruction of intrathoracic lymphatic structures. Pleural fluid cytology and closed pleural biopsy are most often nondiagnostic. Because nearly all patients with pleural effusions due to AIDS and Kaposi's sarcoma are homosexual men with cutaneous sarcomatous lesions, these clinical findings are important clues to diagnosing the etiology of the pleural effusion.

Tuberculous pleurisy is considered to be a manifestation of primary tuberculosis, and its epidemiology is similar to that of pulmonary tuberculosis in general. The peak incidence is in patients less than 45 years of age. Tuberculous pleurisy can result from either a hypersensitivity reaction to a few organisms that enter the pleural space from a subpleural region of pulmonary infection or from direct infection of pleural membrane. Although parenchymal sites of infection are often radiographically inapparent, many patients have histopathologic evidence of lung infection on lung biopsy or autopsy specimens.

The presence of HIV infection appears to alter the clinical presentation of tuberculous pleural effusions. A recent series from New York indicates that patients with tuberculous pleurisy and HIV infection are younger (mean age 38 years) than patients without AIDS (52 years). Patients with HIV disease are also more likely to have negative tuberculin skin tests (59% vs. 24%), positive pleural fluid demonstration of acid-fast organisms (69% vs. 21%), and positive histopathologic examinations of pleural biopsy specimens for acid-fast organisms (53% vs. 23%) compared to patients without HIV disease. The pleural fluid cellular and chemical profile and the likelihood of finding pleural granulomas on pleural biopsy specimens are similar between these two patient populations. The increased load of acid-fast organisms in the pleural space of patients with HIV disease reflects their impaired immune response in that tuberculous pleurisy in the previously healthy host reflects a vigorous immunologic response to a small number of tubercle bacilli.

The occurrence of a pleural effusion in a patient with HIV infection requires a careful evaluation of an extensive differential diagnosis to determine the underlying etiology. Tuberculosis should be specifically considered, however, in patients presenting with an unexplained lymphocyte-predominant exudative pleural effusion even in the absence of a positive tuberculin skin test. A nondiagnostic thoracentesis should be followed by a closed pleural biopsy to search for granulomas and acid-fast organisms. A closed pleural biopsy has a yield of approximately 75% for the diagnosis of tuberculous pleurisy; the yield increases to 90% if a second sample is obtained. If the pleural biopsy is negative, treatment should be initiated empirically if the clinical picture is strongly suggestive of tuberculosis.

The present patient's pleural fluid did not demonstrate tubercle bacilli. He underwent a pleural biopsy that demonstrated caseating granulomas. The patient was discharged from the hospital on multidrug antituberculous chemotherapy.

Clinical Pearls

1. Although common entities, such as bacterial pneumonia and tuberculosis, are frequent causes of pleural effusion in patients with AIDS, more obscure etiologies, such as *Pneumocystis carinii, Cryptococcus neoformans* and *Histoplasma capsulatum* must also be considered.

2. A negative tuberculin test should not dissuade the clinician from considering tuberculosis in a patient with characteristic pleural fluid findings, especially if the patient has HIV disease.

3. Patients with HIV disease are also more likely to have negative tuberculin skin tests (59% vs. 24%), pleural fluid demonstration of acid-fast organisms (69% vs. 21%), and positive histopathologic examinations of pleural biopsy specimens for acid-fast organisms (53% vs. 23%) compared to patients without HIV disease.

REFERENCES

1. O'Brien RF, Cohn DL. Serosanguinous pleural effusion in AIDS-associated Kaposi's sarcoma. Chest 1989;96:460–466.
2. Joseph J, Strange C, Sahn SA. Pleural effusion in hospitalized patients with AIDS. Ann Intern Med 1993;118:856–859.
3. Relkin F, Aranda C, Garay S, et al. Pleural tuberculosis and HIV infection. Chest 1994; 105: 1338–1341.

PATIENT 28

A 52-year-old man with a left upper lobe infiltrate and vocal cord nodules

A 52-year-old man presented with a 3-month history of hoarseness and a nonproductive cough. He denied fevers, night sweats, dyspnea, dysphagia, and odynophagia. His medical history was significant for insulin-dependent diabetes. He had smoked 2 packs of cigarettes per day for over 30 years.

Physical Examination: Normal.

Laboratory Findings: CBC and electrolytes: normal. Chest radiograph: left upper lobe infiltrate. Tuberculin skin test: 10-mm induration. Sputum: 3 smears negative for acid-fast bacilli.

Hospital Course: Fiberoptic bronchoscopy was performed. Two small nodules were observed on the right vocal cord, but were not biopsied. Transbronchial biopsy of the left upper lobe revealed chronic inflammation and fibrosis without granuloma or malignant cells. An otolaryngologist was consulted.

Question: What is the most likely relationship between the vocal cord lesions and the pulmonary disease in this patient?

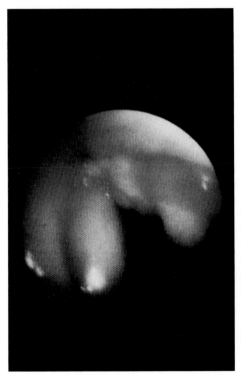 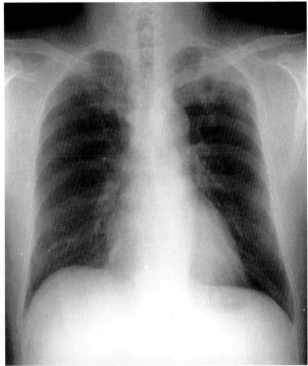

Diagnosis: Tuberculosis with laryngeal and pulmonary involvement.

Discussion: Although recent publications describe laryngeal involvement as a rare manifestation of tuberculosis, autopsy series from the earlier part of the century describe finding laryngeal tuberculosis in one-third to one-half of patients who died of pulmonary tuberculosis. The dramatic change in the incidence of laryngeal tuberculosis is most likely related to the impact that antituberculosis chemotherapy has had on reducing the incidence of the advanced, bilateral cavitary pulmonary tuberculosis almost always associated with laryngeal tuberculosis in the older studies. This association, in combination with the observation that laryngeal tuberculosis usually involved the posterior aspect of the larynx, led investigators to speculate that laryngeal tuberculosis was caused by bacilli-laden sputum pooling in the larynx of prostrate patients. An alternative explanation is that infection of laryngeal structures occurs by hematogenous dissemination. Patients with laryngeal tuberculosis are among the most infectious of patients with tuberculosis.

A recent series of 16 patients reflects the typical presentation of laryngeal tuberculosis in the modern era. Although the majority of patients had pulmonary disease, only one-third had cavities and one-fifth had normal chest radiographs, and no predominance of posterior laryngeal lesions was noted. Other authors have noted a predilection for the anterior laryngeal structures, especially the true vocal cords, and epiglottic involvement is not uncommon.

Hoarseness is a virtually universal complaint of patients with laryngeal tuberculosis. The presence of this symptom, with or without odynophagia or stridor, should raise the suspicion of laryngeal tuberculosis in a patient with typical chest radiographic findings. Laryngoscopic findings are nonspecific and may include edema, ulcerations, nodules, and fungating lesions. While the gross appearance can be mimicked by such entities as papillomatosis, sarcoidosis, Wegener's granulomatosis, and histoplasmosis, the major concern in the differential diagnosis of patients with typical laryngeal lesions is usually squamous cell carcinoma of the larynx. Biopsy of the lesions at laryngoscopy is generally necessary to eliminate this consideration, even if pulmonary tuberculosis has already been demonstrated, because of the reported coexistence of laryngeal tuberculosis and carcinoma in the same patient. Radiographic imaging of the neck, such as CT scan, can delineate the extent of laryngeal involvement in addition to demonstrating the cervical adenopathy often associated with laryngeal tuberculosis, but these findings are nonspecific and generally do not aid in diagnosis.

While the mortality associated with laryngeal tuberculosis in the days before effective treatment of tuberculosis was as high as 70%, with appropriate medical therapy the prognosis is as good as for tuberculosis in general; the laryngeal lesions usually resolve completely within 1–2 months. However, in severe cases, fibrosis of the vocal cords may lead to permanent hoarseness. The presence of stridor may be particularly ominous in this setting, as many patients with this finding require tracheotomy.

The present patient underwent biopsy of his vocal cord abnormalities at laryngoscopy that revealed necrotizing granulomata without evidence of malignancy. Acid-fast stains of the specimens were negative. The patient was placed on standard multidrug antituberculous regimen, with resolution of his symptoms within several weeks. Cultures of sputum and transbronchial biopsy specimens grew *M. tuberculosis* sensitive to all medications. The patient received a total of 6 months of treatment.

Clinical Pearls

1. In the pre-chemotherapeutic era, laryngeal involvement was a common complication of tuberculosis, usually occurring in the setting of advanced, bilateral cavitary lung disease. It was presumably caused by direct inoculation of the larynx by pooled, infectious secretions.

2. Today, laryngeal tuberculosis is a rare entity, and usually is associated with less severe or no lung disease, suggesting local reactivation as a causative mechanism.

3. Suspected laryngeal tuberculosis lesions should be biopsied, even in the setting of known pulmonary tuberculosis, to rule out laryngeal carcinoma.

4. Laryngeal tuberculosis presenting with stridor may require tracheotomy to relieve severe obstruction.

REFERENCES

1. Ramadan HH, Tarazi AE, Baroudy FM. Laryngeal tuberculosis: presentation of 16 cases and review of the literature. J Otolaryngol 1993;22:39–41.
2. Swallow CE, McAdams HP, Colon E. Tuberculosis manifested by a laryngeal mass on CT scans. AJR 1994;163:179–180.

PATIENT 29

**A 73-year-old man with a productive cough and a history of tuberculosis
treated in the sanatorium era**

A 73-year-old smoker presented to the hospital complaining of a worsening cough productive of brown sputum and fever for 4 days. The patient had a history of tuberculosis 45 years earlier that was treated with bed rest in a tuberculosis sanatorium. He had a chronic cough productive of yellow sputum. There was a history of hypertension, atrial fibrillation, and atherosclerotic vascular disease.

Physical Examination: Temperature 101.4°F, respirations 24, pulse 100, blood pressure 140/90 without orthostatic changes. General: elderly thin man in moderate distress. HEENT: normal. Chest: diminished breath sounds and crackles at the bases, bilaterally. Cardiac: irregularly irregular rhythm. Abdomen: normal. Extremities: clubbing. Neurologic: normal.

Laboratory Findings: Hct 38%, WBC 11,600/μl. Electrolytes and liver functions: normal. ABG (room air): pH 7.41, PCO_2 39 mmHg, PO_2 55 mmHg. Chest radiograph: destructive changes and volume loss in the left lung.

Questions: What is the cause of the patient's symptoms? What therapy should be instituted?

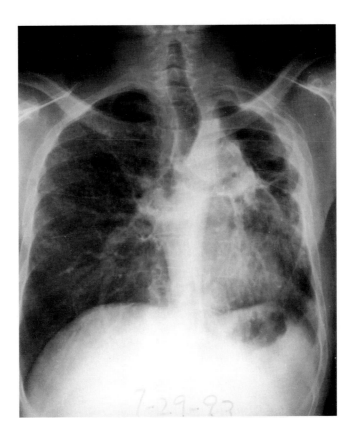

Diagnosis: Bronchiectasis in a patient with prior tuberculosis.

Discussion: Bronchiectasis is an abnormal and permanent dilatation of the airways that most often affects subsegmental bronchi. This condition has long been recognized to be a complication of severe pulmonary tuberculosis. Bronchiectasis is classified on the basis of the radiographic appearance of the dilated segments of bronchi. "Cylindrical" bronchiectasis describes bronchi that are consistently widened throughout an affected segment. "Varicose" bronchiectasis appears as local constrictions that cause an irregular appearance that resembles varicose veins. And "saccular" or "cystic" bronchiectasis refers to dilatations that increase in size toward the lung periphery.

Bronchiectasis results from repeated inflammation of airways, often in a region distal to an airway obstruction, with resultant production of neutrophil elastase that progressively destroys bronchial walls. In adults with tuberculosis, initial obstruction of an airway may occur from drainage of a caseous focus or local penetration of infected lymph nodes into a bronchus. This airway obstruction is followed by progressive inflammation and destruction of distal airways. Bronchiectasis is more likely in patients whose tuberculous disease is far advanced before treatment is initiated or, as in the present patient, who were never treated. Consequently, patients with bronchiectasis related to tuberculosis often have extensive fibrotic and destructive changes of the pulmonary parenchyma related to the underlying tuberculosis. Patients typically have chronic productive coughs and recurrent episodes of airway suppuration due to superinfection of bronchiectatic lung segments. Other causes of bronchiectasis include cystic fibrosis, hypogammaglobulinemia, allergic bronchopulmonary aspergillosis, α-1-antitrypsin deficiency, and syndromes of ciliary dysmotility.

Traditionally, the "gold standard" for diagnosis of bronchiectasis was bronchography. This procedure required the instillation of radiopaque contrast into the tracheobronchial tree for visualization of the distorted bronchial anatomy. In recent years, however, bronchography has been supplanted by high-resolution CT scanning, an easier and more sensitive tool for evaluating the airways. Several groups have defined the CT findings of bronchiec-

tasis: (1) the cystic dilatation of the thick-walled bronchi manifested as strings or clusters of grapes or pearls along the course of the airways; (2) "tram line" appearance of the airways; (3) the "signet ring" sign of fluid-filled cysts around a dilated airway; and (4) "traction bronchiectasis," in which the airways are pulled apart by surrounding fibrotic lung tissue.

Once bronchiectasis has become established, patients are subject to two major complications—bleeding and recurrent pneumonia. The bacteriology of pneumonia in a patient with underlying bronchiectasis includes all of the usual bacterial pathogens, with gram-negative organisms playing a major role in exacerbations. *Pseudomonas aeruginosa* is a particular concern in this patient population. A recent study from Hong Kong pointed out that *Mycobacterium tuberculosis* may also complicate bronchiectasis. Ninety-one consecutive patients with bronchiectasis were evaluated over 9 years, and positive cultures for mycobacteria were found in 12 (13%). Of these, *M. tuberculosis* was isolated in 9/12 patients; the investigators noted that tuberculosis was not strongly suspected on clinical grounds in any of the 9 patients with the disease. Thus, in addition to the usual bacterial pathogens that complicate bronchiectasis, one should remember mycobacteria in a patient who does not respond to antibacterial therapy. More definitive therapy, such as removal of a severely affected region of the lung, is appropriate for patients who have severe and recurrent symptoms in the presence of localized disease.

The present patient presented with a remote history of untreated tuberculosis and recent worsening of his chronic cough associated with fever. This presentation was compatible with reactivation tuberculosis or an exacerbation of underlying bronchiectasis with or without an accompanying pneumonia. The patient was treated with amoxicillin-clavulanic acid with a good clinical response. Sputum cultures subsequently grew *H. influenzae* and were negative for *M. tuberculosis*. Because he had never received drug therapy for tuberculosis and his mycobacterial cultures were negative, he was placed on isoniazid prophylaxis.

Clinical Pearls

1. Bronchiectasis is a relatively common complication of severe or untreated pulmonary tuberculosis.

2. The diagnosis is suggested by the characteristic clinical syndrome and can usually be confirmed by high-resolution CT scanning.

3. Most exacerbations of bronchiectasis are due to bacterial pathogens, including gram-negative organisms; mycobacteria should be suspected in instances where prompt improvement with antibacterial therapy does not occur.

REFERENCES

1. Reid LM. Reduction in bronchial subdivision in bronchiectasis. Thorax 1950;5:233–247.
2. Naidich DP, McCauley DI, Khouri NF, et al. Computed tomography of bronchiectasis. J Comput Assist Tomogr 1982;6:437–444.
3. Westcott JL. Bronchiectasis. Radiol Clin North Am 1991;29:1031–1042.
4. Trucksis M, Swartz MN. Bronchiectasis: a current view. Curr Clin Topics Infect Dis 1991;11:170–205.
5. Chan CH, Ho AK, Chan RC, et al. Mycobacteria as a cause of infective exacerbation in bronchiectasis. Postgrad Med J 1992;68:896–899.

PATIENT 30

A 28-year-old man with HIV infection and 6 months of therapy for pulmonary tuberculosis

A 28-year-old man was referred for evaluation of his treatment for tuberculosis. He was known to be HIV seropositive with a diagnosis of tuberculosis made 7 months previously. He was treated initially with a four-drug regimen, and when susceptibility testing revealed that his isolate was sensitive to all medications, his regimen was adjusted to isoniazid, rifampin, and pyrazinamide. He completed a total of 6 months of therapy. At the time of his visit to the chest clinic, he was without symptoms.

Physical Examination: Vital signs: normal. General: comfortable. Entire examination: normal.

Laboratory Findings: CBC and electrolytes: normal. Chest radiograph: small fibrotic density in the left upper lobe, improved since the patient's initial diagnosis. Initial sputum culture: positive for *M. tuberculosis*. Subsequent sputum cultures: negative for mycobacteria.

Question: Does the patient require further therapy?

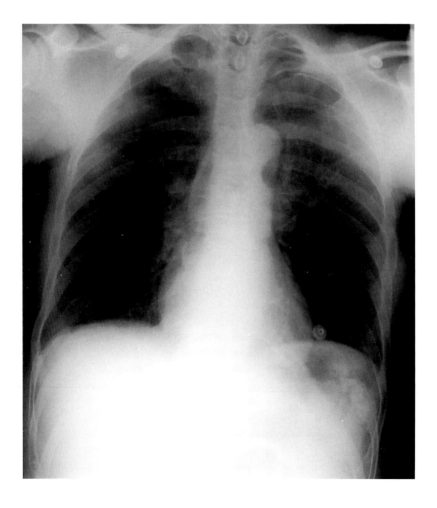

Diagnosis: Adequately treated pulmonary tuberculosis in a patient with AIDS.

Discussion: Tuberculosis is a common and extremely important pulmonary complication of HIV infection. For many years, the Centers for Disease Control and Prevention recognized extrapulmonary tuberculosis as an AIDS-defining illness. More recently with the observed high prevalence of pulmonary tuberculosis in patients with HIV infection, this form of tuberculosis has also been listed as a disorder that defines AIDS in the presence of HIV seropositivity.

Experience with other AIDS-related infections has taught clinicians that recurrence is common if treatment is not continued for a prolonged period or if prophylaxis is not instituted. For example, prolonged therapy for coccidioidomycosis is required to maintain disease suppression, and secondary prophylaxis has shown to be necessary for the management of patients with pneumonia due to *Pneumocystis carinii*. On the basis of these observations, clinicians have had justified concerns that AIDS patients may require specialized considerations in the treatment of even drug-susceptible tuberculosis.

Early reports during the AIDS epidemic suggested that patients with HIV infection treated for tuberculosis were more likely than otherwise normal hosts to have recurrence of their tubercular disease. These observations, however, may have resulted from the use of drug regimens, such as isoniazid, thioacetazone, and streptomycin, which are less effective than regimens that incorporate rifampin. Furthermore, some of these series included patients who were non-compliant with therapy. And finally, studies using restriction fragment length polymorphism analysis to compare the DNA fingerprints of the initial and recurrent *M. tuberculosis* isolates demonstrate that some apparent "recurrences" of tuberculosis actually result from exogenous reinfection.

More recent data suggest that patients with AIDS require no specialized drug regimens for the management of tuberculosis. Current ATS/CDC guidelines state that AIDS patients with pulmonary tuberculosis may receive short-course (including 6 month) therapy. However, patients must be closely followed during treatment both to ensure compliance and to monitor the response to treatment. If there are indications that either of these issues are not proceeding satisfactorily, treatment may need to be prolonged. Currently there are no data to support the continuation of a single drug as secondary prophylaxis after a course of treatment is completed. This practice is potentially dangerous because of the risk of generating resistant strains of *M. tuberculosis*. AIDS patients who have completed a course of therapy, however, should be closely monitored by their physician for disease recurrence or reinfection with a new strain.

The present patient felt well and his records indicated that he had complied with an adequate therapeutic regimen. He was not retreated with any additional drugs. He was followed carefully by his physicians and maintained on prophylactic therapy for the nontuberculous AIDS-related infections.

Clinical Pearls

1. AIDS patients with pulmonary tuberculosis with drug susceptible strains can, in general, be treated with the identical short-course chemotherapy regimens used in HIV-negative persons.

2. Apparent relapses in AIDS patients are often due to inadequate initial therapy or to exogenous reinfection with a new strain of mycobacteria.

3. Secondary prophylaxis is not recommended for AIDS patients who have completed an effective course of chemotherapy for pulmonary tuberculosis.

REFERENCES

1. Small PM, Schecter GF, Goodman PC, et al. Treatment of tuberculosis in patients with advanced human immunodeficiency virus infection. N Engl J Med 1991;324:289–294.
2. Small PM, Shafer RW, Hopewell PC, et al. Exogenous reinfection with multidrug-resistant *Mycobacterium tuberculosis* in patients with advanced HIV infection. N Engl J Med 1993;328:1137–1144.
3. Hawken M, Nunn P, Gathua S, et al. Increased recurrence of tuberculosis in HIV-1-infected patients in Kenya. Lancet 1993;342:332–337.
4. Jones BE, Otaya M, Antoniskis D, et al. A prospective evaluation of antituberculous therapy in patients with human immunodeficiency virus infection. Am J Respir Crit Care Med 1994;150:1499–1503.

PATIENT 31

An 18-year-old pregnant woman with a positive tuberculin skin test and an abnormal chest radiograph

An 18-year-old woman in the sixth month of an uncomplicated pregnancy presented with a positive tuberculin test with 14 mm of induration and an abnormal chest radiograph. The patient denied fever, chills, cough, sputum production, night sweats, or weight loss. There was no known contact with anyone with tuberculosis.

Physical Examination: Vital signs: normal. General: comfortable. HEENT: normal. Chest: diminished breath sounds with egophony at the left upper lobe. Cardiac: normal heart sounds without murmurs or rubs. Abdomen: gravid, otherwise normal. Extremities: normal. Neurologic: normal.

Laboratory Findings: CBC, electrolytes, liver function tests: normal. Chest radiograph (shown below): consolidation of the left upper lobe, with air bronchograms. Induced sputum: negative for acid-fast bacilli.

Question: What diagnostic and therapeutic interventions should be initiated?

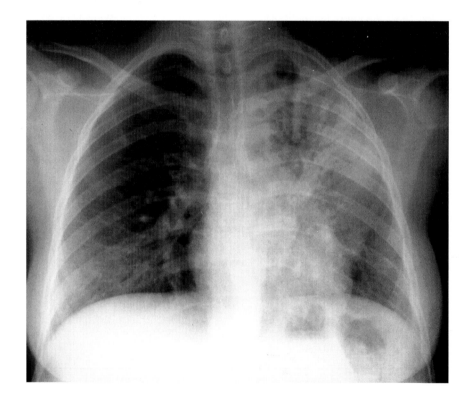

Diagnosis: Active pulmonary tuberculosis in a pregnant woman.

Discussion: As a consequence of the increasing prevalence of tuberculosis in the United States since 1985, recent public health data indicate that tuberculosis among pregnant women is also on the rise. Previous concepts have suggested that pregnancy may increase the risk of reactivation of latent tuberculous infections. Current thinking, however, concludes that the natural history of tuberculosis is affected little if at all by pregnancy.

The increasing prevalence of tuberculosis in pregnant women and the risks of infection in newborn infants, however, warrant careful adherence to public health recommendations in caring for women of childbearing age at risk for this disease. First, in high-risk groups, tuberculin screening is now a routine part of prenatal care. Second, every positive tuberculin test that is detected during prenatal screening must be followed up to exclude the possibility of active tuberculosis. This evaluation should include a chest radiograph because pregnant patients with active tuberculosis may be relatively asymptomatic or have symptoms ascribed to the pregnancy. For instance, dyspnea accompanying tuberculosis may be attributed to the physiologic effects of a gravid uterus in the second and third trimester.

If the tuberculin skin test is positive and the chest radiograph abnormal, the diagnosis of active tuberculosis must be vigorously pursued and promptly treated if present. If the diagnosis and treatment are delayed, a considerable risk of postnatal transmission to the newborn infant exists if the mother remains untreated at the time of delivery and during the early postpartum period. Furthermore, congenital tuberculosis—transplacental infection of the fetus—can rarely occur. Although still controversial, recent data from a single patient series suggest that untreated tuberculosis in the mother increases the risk for premature delivery by twofold, low birth weight, and perinatal mortality.

The diagnosis of tuberculosis is pursued in a pregnant woman in a similar manner as with any other patient. Sputum smears and cultures have an identical diagnostic yield as in other patient populations. Although pregnancy does not constitute a contraindication to diagnostic bronchoscopy in patients with negative sputum evaluations, care must be taken to ensure adequate oxygenation of both the patient and the fetus during the procedure.

Once a decision to treat active tuberculosis in a pregnant woman is made, therapy should be promptly instituted so that the patient will not be infectious at the time of delivery. Isoniazid, rifampin, and ethambutol are currently recommended by the American Thoracic Society (ATS) for use in pregnancy. The European Respiratory Society also recommends pyrazinamide, but the absence of safety data for its use in pregnancy has caused the ATS and the Centers for Disease Control and Prevention to recommend avoiding its use. If the patient is infected with a pan-sensitive strain, an excellent outcome for both mother and infant can be expected. The presence of multidrug-resistant tuberculosis, however, presents special challenges. Streptomycin is contraindicated in pregnancy because of the risk of fetal ototoxicity, and the quinolones should be avoided as well because of concerns about arthropathy in the developing fetus. These contraindications severely limit therapeutic options and may, in some patients, force the use of agents that have limited safety data for their use in pregnancy. This situation should be carefully discussed with the patient and her husband.

Sputum smears from the present patient were negative and she underwent fiberoptic bronchoscopy. Initial bronchoscopic specimens were negative but because of the high clinical suspicion for tuberculosis, she was discharged on a drug regimen that included isoniazid, rifampin, and ethambutol. The initial sputum sputum subsequently grew *M. tuberculosis,* sensitive to all drugs. She went on to deliver a healthy full-term infant.

Clinical Pearls

1. High-risk patients should be screened with tuberculin skin tests during pregnancy and all positive tests should be evaluated with a chest radiograph, performed with appropriate abdominal shielding.

2. When sputum smears are negative in a patient with suspected tuberculosis, the risks and benefits of bronchoscopy should be weighed against the risks and benefits of empiric therapy.

3. Isoniazid, rifampin, and ethambutol are recommended for initial therapy in pregnant patients with active tuberculosis. If aminoglycosides, quinolones, or other second-line agents need to be used, the patient, spouse, and physician should carefully discuss the therapeutic options and risks to the mother and infant of untreated tuberculosis.

REFERENCES

1. Wilson EA, Thelin TJ, Dilts PV. Tuberculosis complicated by pregnancy. Am J Obstet Gynecol 1973;115:526.
2. Good JT, Iseman MD, Davidson PT, et al. Tuberculosis in association with pregnancy. Am J Obstet Gynecol 1981;140:492–498.
3. Jana N, Vasishta K, Jindal SK, et al. Perinatal outcome in pregnancies complicated by pulmonary tuberculosis. Int J Gynecol Obstet 1994;44:119–124.
4. Carter EJ, Mates S. Tuberculosis during pregnancy: the Rhode Island experience. Chest 1994;1466–1471.
5. Margono F, Mroueh J, Garely A, et al. Resurgence of active tuberculosis among pregnant women. Obstet Gynecol 1994;83:911–914.

PATIENT 32

A 48-year-old woman with thrombocytopenia during treatment for tuberculosis

A 48-year-old woman presented for routine follow-up 2 months after starting drug therapy for tuberculous mediastinal lympadenopathy. Aspiration of the lymph nodes had demonstrated *Mycobacterium tuberculosis* sensitive to all drugs. Her original symptoms of fever and cough had resolved on a regimen that consisted of isoniazid, rifampin, pyrazinamide, and ethambutol. The patient had tested negative for HIV at the time of her diagnosis and denied risk factors for HIV disease, use of other medications, or alcohol ingestion. Her hemogram had been normal when she started antituberculous drug therapy.

Physical Examination: Vital signs: normal. General: comfortable. Chest: clear. Lymph nodes: nonpalpable. Cardiac: no murmurs. Abdomen: no organomegaly. Extremities: normal.

Laboratory Findings: Hct 39%, WBC 7,000/µl, platelets 23,000/µl. Liver function tests: normal. Sputum smear: negative for acid-fast organisms. Stool exam for occult blood: negative. Chest radiograph: resolving mediastinal adenopathy.

Question: What is the most likely cause of thrombocytopenia in this patient?

Diagnosis: Rifampin-induced thrombocytopenia.

Discussion: Rifampin represented a major advance in the management of tuberculosis when it was first introduced into clinical practice in 1972. It provided such effective activity against *Mycobacterium tuberculosis* that short-course chemotherapeutic regimens became a clinical possibility. Furthermore, rifampin is relatively well tolerated in most patients with a low incidence of adverse drug reactions. When side effects to rifampin do occur, they usually affect the gastrointestinal tract, liver, and skin. Nausea, anorexia, and diarrhea are the most common gastrointestinal manifestations of rifampin toxicity but rarely affect patients so severely to require the discontinuation of the drug. These side effects can be lessened if patients take rifampin 2 hours after meals. Ingestion of rifampin with meals should be avoided, however, because of decreased drug absorption.

Drug-induced hepatitis represents a more serious complication of rifampin therapy. The frequency of this complication is unclear, but appears to be quite low, even when rifampin is combined with other hepatotoxic agents such as isoniazid or pyrazinamide. A recent meta-analysis, however, suggests that the combination of isoniazid and rifampin does have a minimally increased, albeit low, risk of hepatitis compared to the use of isoniazid in regimens that do not contain rifampin. It is unknown whether isoniazid has a synergistic or additive effect in increasing the incidence of rifampin-induced hepatitis. Because drug-induced hepatitis can be severe in some patients, the onset of any symptoms compatible with this diagnosis in patients on rifampin-containing regimens should prompt the determination of liver function tests.

Thrombocytopenia is fortunately an infrequent complication of rifampin therapy. Isoniazid and ethambutol may also produce this complication but much less commonly than rifampin. Thrombocytopenia appears to belong to a group of immune-mediated side effects induced by rifampin. Other immune-mediated complications, which generally only occur at doses (20 mg/kg) rarely used in clinical practice, include a severe influenza-like reaction, hemolytic anemia, renal failure, and respiratory failure. Any of these complications mandate immediate discontinuation of the drug and consideration of treatment with corticosteroids. Patients who suffer these life-threatening reactions should not receive rifampin again. Interestingly, mild allergic reactions may occur in patients receiving intermittent (e.g., twice weekly) therapy, or in those whose treatment course is interrupted by periods of noncompliance. Although the allergic reactions in these patients may resolve if rifampin is taken daily, a trial of desensitization is often effective and probably should be attempted.

Most clinicians are aware that rifampin imparts an orange color to all body fluids, but they must remember to warn patients to expect this potentially frightening phenomenon. The only clinical significance of this effect is that soft contact lenses will be permanently stained by orange tears, even after a single dose.

Important indirect side effects of rifampin are related to its potent induction of hepatic microsomal enzymes, which greatly increases the rate of clearance of other drugs metabolized by these enzymes. Close monitoring of the effectiveness of medications, such as oral anticoagulants, contraceptives, corticosteroids, methadone, oral hypoglycemics, ketoconazole, cyclosporine, quinidine, and digitoxin, must be initiated when these medications are given in conjunction with rifampin. Most patients treated with rifampin will require increases in the dosages of these other medications. Breakthrough bleeding and even pregnancies may occur in women taking oral contraceptives because of the enzyme induction effects of rifampin. Women taking rifampin should be advised to use alternative methods of birth control.

The present patient was called back to the clinic the next day when her platelet count results became available. A repeat platelet count was 5,000/µl. The patient was hospitalized, antituberculous therapy was discontinued, and platelet transfusions and corticosteroids were administered. No bleeding complications occurred. Ten days later the platelet count had risen to 50,000/µl and normalized thereafter. Isoniazid and ethambutol were restarted, and the patient completed an 18-month course of therapy without further complications.

Clinical Pearls

1. Thrombocytopenia rarely occurs in patients being treated for tuberculosis. When present, it is most often attributable to rifampin.

2. Because rifampin is a powerful inducer of hepatic microsomal enzymes, interactions with drugs such as oral anticoagulants, corticosteroids, methadone, oral hypoglycemics, ketoconazole, cyclosporine, quinidine, and digitoxin may necessitate increased doses of these medications. Close monitoring of effectiveness of these drugs during rifampin therapy is advised.

3. Women who use oral contraceptives should be advised to employ alternative means of birth control while taking rifampin.

4. Mild allergic reactions to rifampin may be overcome by desensitization to the drug.

REFERENCES

1. Baciewicz AM, Self TH. Rifampin drug interactions. Arch Intern Med 1984; 144:1667–1671.
2. Lee CH, Lee CJ. Thrombocytopenia—a rare but potentially serious side effect of initial daily and interrupted use of rifampin. Chest 1989;96:202–203.
3. Steele MA, Burk RF, DesPrez RM. Toxic hepatitis with isoniazid and rifampin: a meta-analysis. Chest 1991;99:465–471.
4. Matz J, Borish LC, Routes JM, Rossenwasser LJ. Oral desensitization to rifampin and ethambutol in mycobacterial disease. Am J Respir Crit Care Med 1994;149:815–817.

PATIENT 33

A 40-year-old man with paratracheal adenopathy

A 40-year-old man with a history of intravenous drug abuse presented with fever, night sweats, and malaise of several weeks' duration. He denied weight loss, cough, or dyspnea. The patient had never been tested for HIV and recalled a negative tuberculin skin test a year earlier. He was homeless and had intermittently spent time in the shelter system.

Physical Examination: Temperature 103°F, pulse 108, respirations 20. General: chronically ill and disheveled. Skin: needle marks on both arms. Lymph nodes: generalized "shotty" lymphadenopathy.

Laboratory Findings: Hct 32%, WBC 3600/μl. HIV test: positive. CD4+ cell count: 81/μl. Chest radiograph: widened right paratracheal stripe. Chest CT: enlarged right paratracheal lymph node with decreased attenuation centrally; no parenchymal abnormalities. Sputum: multiple smears negative for acid-fast bacilli.

Question: What is the best approach to diagnosis in this patient?

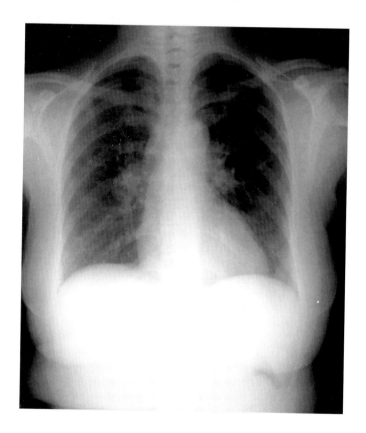

Diagnosis: Mediastinal tuberculous lymphadenitis

Discussion: Patients with HIV-infection who develop intrathoracic tuberculosis most often present with atypical radiographic patterns compared to the immunocompetent host. Although some patients in the early stages of AIDS may develop tuberculosis with upper lobe cavitary infiltrates typical for reactivation disease, the majority of patients have radiographic findings similar to those that occur in patients with primary tuberculosis. These findings include pleural effusions, mediastinal and hilar adenopathy, and miliary nodules. Patients with AIDS who develop tuberculosis may also present with a normal chest radiograph or diffuse interstitial infiltrates, although these findings are uncommon.

The presence of intrathoracic adenopathy in patients with HIV infection presents a differential diagnosis that includes lymphoma, Kaposi's sarcoma, and various fungal infections in addition to mycobacterial disease. In this setting, a chest CT with contrast can assist in determining the likelihood of tuberculous lymphadenitis. Tuberculous nodes may often appear massively enlarged with a central area of low density surrounded by a peripheral rim of contrast enhancement. This pattern usually does not occur in patients with lymphoma, but has been reported in various fungal diseases. A similar CT appearance may also develop in patients with lung cancer and malignant lymph nodes undergoing central necrosis.

Even in the presence of suggestive CT findings, patients with HIV disease and mediastinal adenopathy should undergo diagnostic sampling of the enlarged lymph nodes for histopathologic and microbiologic studies. Most surgeons would prefer to avoid invasive surgical procedures, such as mediastinoscopy or mediastinotomy, in the setting of nonmalignant disease. Less invasive procedures include percutaneous needle aspiration and fiberoptic bronchoscopy (FOB) with transbronchial needle aspiration (TBNA) of parabronchial and paratracheal nodes. The latter technique was originally developed to sample intrathoracic lymph nodes for staging patients with lung cancer. Lymph nodes in the hilar, subcarinal, paratracheal, and aorticopulmonary window are accessible by these techniques. A recently developed 19g needle allows the sampling of sufficiently large core specimens to establish a specific diagnosis in patients with nonmalignant disorders. In addition to its efficacy in diagnosing patients with sarcoidosis, TBNA has been used to confirm the diagnosis of tuberculous lymphadenitis, as well as lymphadenitis due to nontuberculous mycobacteria such as *M. avium-intracellulare* and *M. fortuitum*. In these clinical settings, TBNA has a diagnostic yield for mycobacterial infections of 75%. It is a safe procedure that has a lower complication rate than fiberoptic bronchoscopy with transbronchial biopsy.

CT-guided transthoracic needle aspiration biopsy is an alternative, minimally invasive, and safe technique for diagnosing tuberculous mediastinal lymphadenopathy in patients with HIV disease. The diagnostic yield and safety of this technique are comparable to TBNA in patients with intrathoracic tuberculous lymphadenitis. The success of TBNA and transthoracic needle aspiration biopsy depends greatly on the experience of the operator.

The present patient underwent fiberoptic bronchoscopy with TBNA of the right paratracheal lymph node. Poorly formed necrotizing granulomata were found, and acid-fast organisms were seen. The patient was treated with isoniazid, rifampin, pyrazinamide, and ethambutol. Although cultures of aspirated material from the TBNA did not grow organisms, the patient's symptoms resolved and the chest radiograph several months later was normal.

Clinical Pearls

1. Chest radiograph findings in patients with tuberculosis and HIV infection, particularly in those with AIDS, often resemble the findings in immunocompetent patients with primary tuberculosis.

2. In patients with HIV infection, the finding on chest CT of low-density intrathoracic lymph nodes, with or without peripheral contrast enhancement, is highly suggestive of tuberculosis.

3. The diagnosis of tuberculosis and other mycobacterial infections can be made readily and safely by sampling enlarged mediastinal and hilar lymph nodes using TBNA during bronchoscopy.

4. CT-guided transthoracic needle aspiration biopsy is a useful alternative to diagnose intrathoracic tuberculous lymphadenitis.

REFERENCES

1. Barnes PF, Bloch AB, Davidson PT, Snider DE. Tuberculosis in patients with human immunodeficiency virus infection. N Engl J Med 1991;324:1644–50.
2. Pastores SM, Naidich DP, Aranda CP, et al. Intrathoracic adenopathy associated with pulmonary tuberculosis in patients with human immunodeficiency virus infection. Chest 1993;103:1433–37.
3. Harkin TJ, Karp J, Ciotoli C, et al. Transbronchial needle aspiration in the diagnosis of mediastinal mycobacterial infection. Am Rev Respir Dis 1993;147:A801.
4. Wang KP. Staging of bronchogenic carcinoma by bronchoscopy. Chest 1994;106:588–593.
5. Khan J, Akhtar M, von Sinner WN, et al. CT-guided fine needle aspiration biopsy in the diagnosis of mediastinal tuberculosis. Chest 1994;106:1329–1332.

PATIENT 34

A 30-year-old HIV-infected man with cutaneous anergy

A 30-year-old man presented to his physician for tuberculosis screening. He was infected with HIV and had a previous history of intravenous drug abuse. There was no history of previous opportunistic infections. The patient was asymptomatic and denied recent contact with persons with active tuberculosis.

Physical Examination: Vital signs: normal. General: comfortable. The remainder of the physical examination was normal.

Laboratory Findings: CBC, electrolytes, liver function tests: normal. CD4+ cell count: 200/μl. Tuberculin skin test: no induration at 48 or 72 hours. Anergy testing: no response to candida, mumps, or tetanus. Chest radiograph: normal.

Questions: How should the possibility of tuberculosis infection be evaluated in this patient? What therapy, if any, should be given?

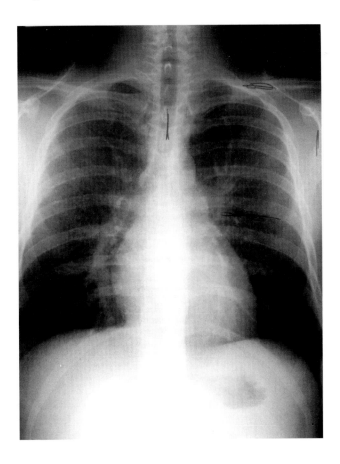

Diagnosis: Cutaneous anergy in a patient with HIV infection at risk for tuberculosis.

Discussion: It is widely appreciated that patients with HIV infection are at high risk for developing active tuberculosis if they have latent tuberculosis infection. Furthermore, it is known that much of the tuberculous disease in this population occurs as a result of recent transmission: the time between infection and development of disease in AIDS patients may be as short as 1 month. In view of these risks, tuberculin screening and isoniazid preventive therapy are of great importance in the HIV-infected population.

Any HIV-infected person with a positive tuberculin test (5 mm or more of induration) should receive isoniazid preventive therapy for 12 months, unless such therapy had previously been given. This recommendation stands regardless of the patient's age, CD4+ cell count, or length of time that the skin test has been known to be positive. Considerable evidence establishes that isoniazid preventive therapy is effective in this patient population. However, a more difficult management problem arises in patients who have cutaneous anergy and thereby have lost the ability to be defined as tuberculin skin test positive or negative.

In approaching this problem, accumulating clinical data demonstrate that the risk of developing active tuberculosis in anergic HIV-infected patients with known or suspected exposure to tuberculosis approaches or equals that of patients with HIV disease who are tuberculin skin test positive. One group of investigators found that the rate of developing active tuberculosis among anergic, HIV-seropositive drug abusers (6.6 cases/100 person years) was not statistically different from HIV-seropositive drug abusers with positive tuberculin tests who were not receiving isoniazid preventive therapy (9.7 cases/100 person-years). No instances of active tuberculosis developed in HIV-seropositive, tuberculin-skin-test positive patients who had received a year of isoniazid preventive therapy. Similarly, another study found the case rate for development of active tuberculosis to be 12.4/100 person-years for anergic, HIV-seropositive patients compared to 10/100 person-years for untreated HIV-positive, tuberculin-skin-test positive individuals. These investigators also determined that this risk applied almost entirely to those patients who had become HIV infected through the intravenous abuse of illicit drugs. This observation corresponds to the well-known risk for tuberculosis infection among certain segments of the population, such as injection drug users, who may find themselves in congregate settings, such as prisons or shelters, where infection can easily spread from person to person.

The above information suggests several strategies for diagnosis and treatment of anergic HIV-infected patients who may be infected with tuberculosis. One approach might be to follow such patients clinically with interval chest radiographs to detect early pulmonary tuberculosis. Even if totally effective in the early detection of tuberculosis, however, this strategy would not allow for the prevention of active disease. Increasing evidence indicates that active tuberculosis may actually accelerate the natural history of HIV infection, so that the "watchful waiting" strategy may result in significant morbidity in HIV-infected patients.

Alternatively, isoniazid could be given for 1 year to any person with HIV infection. This strategy was first suggested as the result of a decision analysis that weighed the risks and benefits of isoniazid preventive therapy in seropositive persons. Using estimates of both the incidence of isoniazid hepatitis and the chance of developing active tuberculosis, the authors found conditions favorable for administering isoniazid, regardless of the tuberculin skin test result, to all HIV seropositive intravenous drug users. The only exception were black women, who for unclear reasons had an unfavorable risk/benefit profile in this analysis. Although resting on generally sound assumptions, this study is limited by its theoretical nature and the absence of empiric supporting data.

A third strategy is to perform anergy testing with several antigens (candida, mumps, trichophyton, tetanus) if initial tuberculin skin testing is negative. If the patient is indeed anergic, the physician would then consider the tuberculin skin test as a possible false negative, and isoniazid preventive therapy would be given. Although anergy testing is a complex and poorly understood phenomenon, the rate of development of active tuberculosis among anergic HIV-infected injection drug users supports this approach to prophylaxis in this population. Consequently, recent recommendations encourage the initiation of isoniazid parophylaxis to HIV-infected persons in the presence of anergy if they appear to be at high risk for tuberculous infection. Risk factors include injection use of illicit drugs, residence in a shelter or other congregate settings, and close contact with an individual with tuberculosis.

The present patient was prescribed isoniazid preventive therapy to be taken for 1 year. He was compliant with the prophylactic regimen during the duration of drug treatment.

Clinical Pearls

1. The incidence of cutaneous anergy rises sharply among HIV-infected persons as the CD4+ cell count falls.

2. HIV-infected patients with cutaneous anergy and a history of injection drug abuse have a similar incidence of contracting active tuberculosis compared to HIV-infected patients with a positive tuberculin skin test.

3. Existing data support the performance of anergy testing in HIV-infected, tuberculin-negative persons. Isoniazid prophylaxis should be initiated for those found to be anergic if additional clinical risk factors for tuberculosis exist.

4. Some clinicians recommend that prophylactic isoniazid be given to all HIV-infected persons with cutaneous anergy. Little empiric evidence exists, however, to support this recommendation.

REFERENCES

1. Jordan TJ, Lewit EM, Montgomery RL, Reichman LB. Isoniazid as preventive therapy in HIV-infected intravenous drug abusers: a decision analysis. JAMA 1991;265:2987–2991.
2. Selwyn PA, Schell BM, Alcalbes P, et al. High risk of active tuberculosis in HIV-infected drug users with cutaneous anergy. JAMA 1992;268:504–509.
3. Moreno S, Baraia-Etxaburu J, Bouza E, et al. Risk for developing tuberculosis among anergic patients infected with HIV. Ann Intern Med 1993;119:194–198.

PATIENT 35

A 36-year-old man with fever, headache, and an abnormal chest radiograph

A 36-year-old man presented complaining of dyspnea, fever, and a headache for 1 week. He denied other pulmonary or systemic symptoms. The patient had been previously well and had arrived in the United States from Morocco 3 months earlier. He worked in a bakery and had no history of tobacco use or known contact with persons with tuberculosis.

Physical Examination: Temperature 102.4°F, pulse 108, respirations 22, blood pressure 130/76. General: acutely ill, moderate respiratory distress. HEENT: meningismus noted. Chest: minimal bibasilar fine rales. Cardiac: normal heart hounds without murmurs or rubs. Abdomen: normal. Extremities: normal. Neurologic: normal.

Laboratory Findings: CBC, electrolytes, liver function tests, and coagulation profile: normal. Chest radiograph: multiple 2–3-mm nodules diffusely throughout all lung fields. Lumbar puncture: opening pressure 16 cmH$_2$O, protein 250 mg/dl, glucose 80 mg/dl, nucleated cell count 180/μl, 75% lymphocytes. Acid-fast smears of sputum and cerebrospinal fluid: negative. A tuberculin skin test was placed.

Question: What therapy should be instituted in this patient?

Diagnosis: Tuberculous meningitis in a patient with disseminated (miliary) tuberculosis.

Discussion: Tuberculous involvement of the central nervous system represents one of the most severe manifestions of the disease. The three major forms of this condition include meningitis, tuberculoma, and spinal abscess. Of these, meningitis is the most common.

Tuberculous meningitis occurs most often in children less than 4 years of age. Recent reports, however, indicate an increasing incidence of this disorder in adults who have AIDS. Central nervous system tuberculosis still represents only 5% of cases of extrapulmonary tuberculosis.

The diagnosis of tuberculous meningitis should be suspected in any patient presenting with a headache and meningismus with a cerebrospinal fluid (CSF) profile of an elevated protein concentration and a predominance of lymphocytes. Any chest radiographic evidence of tuberculosis should further increase clinical suspicion of tuberculous meningitis. Other manifestations of this condition include focal neurologic findings, which usually present as cranial nerve abnormalities as a result of the predominantly basilar location of the meningitis. Chest radiographs will be abnormal in at least half of patients with tuberculous meningitis. These radiographic findings may be one of the most important clues to the diagnosis because the neurologic signs and symptoms are often mild or nonspecific in a substantial proportion of patients.

The CSF profile is nonspecific but highly suggestive of tuberculous meningitis in the right clinical setting. Lymphocytosis is a predominant finding, with the total nucleated cells ranging from 100 to 1000 cell/μl. The protein is typically elevated; patients who develop a block to CSF flow may have extraordinarily high concentrations of fluid protein. The glucose concentration is not as low as in bacterial meningitis. Unfortunately, acid-fast smears of CSF are positive in only 10–20% of patients and seldom suffice to establish a definitive diagnosis before the inititation of therapy.

Recent investigations indicate that two new tests—the detection of mycobacterial fatty acids and the polymerase chain reaction (PCR) assay—may provide important advances in establishing an early diagnosis of tuberculous meningitis. Detection of mycobacterial fatty or carboxylic acids (most often tuberculostearic acid) using gas-liquid chromatography (GLC) has been shown by several groups to have a sensitivity of 95–100% and a specificity of 90%. Unfortunately, GLC is a cumbersome and expensive technique that is available at very few medical centers. Diagnosis by PCR may be a more practical method. This technique is extremely sensitive for the detection of small numbers of acid-fast organisms. It can amplify and establish the presence of as few as one copy of genomic DNA from a single bacterium in a submitted patient specimen within 6 hours. Recent studies using a commercially available PCR test demonstrate that analysis of sputum from patients with active tuberculosis has the same positivity rate (58%) as sputum cultures (56%). Although PCR presents considerable promise, there are no large patient series to date that establish the sensitivity and specificity of PCR for the diagnosis of tuberculous meningitis.

Once a presumptive diagnosis of tuberculous meningitis is made, therapy should be instituted without delay. Of the first-line chemotherapeutic agents, all except ethambutol have good to excellent penetration into the meninges, particularly when inflammation is present. The major debate in the treatment of tuberculous meningitis concerns the use of corticosteroids. Generally acceptable indications for steroid use include a very high CSF protein concentration (a finding associated with arachnoiditis and the possibility of spinal fluid block), cerebral edema, or focal neurologic (most often cranial nerve) findings. In children with the disease, more liberal use of corticosteroids may be justified, because there is evidence that their use may decrease long-term sequelae, such as hearing loss.

The present patient was started on a regimen of isoniazid, rifampin, pyrazinamide, and streptomycin. Neurologic consultants advised against the initiation of corticosteroids considering that they were not necessary in the absence of the usual indications. A transbronchial biopsy detected numerous granulomas without acid-fast organisms. Eventually, the transbronchial biopsy specimen and the CSF grew *Mycobacterium tuberculosis*. The patient made an uneventful recovery without neurologic sequelae.

Clinical Pearls

1. Tuberculous meningitis should be considered in any patient with meningeal irritation and a chest radiograph suggestive of tuberculosis.

2. Characteristic CSF findings of high protein and lymphocytosis should also suggest tuberculous meningitis.

3. If readily available, tuberculostearic acid assay and PCR performed on the CSF provide an early diagnosis.

4. Accepted indications for steroid use include cranial nerve findings, an extremely elevated CSF protein, and cerebral edema.

REFERENCES

1. Brooks JB, Daneshvar MI, Haberberger RL, et al. Rapid diagnosis of tuberculous meningitis by frequency-pulsed electron capture gas-liquid chromatography detection of carboxylic acids in cerebrospinal fluid. J Clin Microbiol 1990;28:989–997.
2. Humphries M. The management of tuberculous meningitis. Thorax 1992;47:577–581.
3. Berenguer J, Moreno S, Laguna F, et al. Tuberculous meningitis in patients infected with the human immunodeficiency virus. N Engl J Med 1992;326:668–672.
4. Kent SJ, Crowe SM, Yung A, et al. Tuberculous meningitis: a 30-year review. Clin Infect Dis 1993;17:987–994.
5. Chin DP, Yajko DM, Hadley, WK, et al. Clinical utility of a commercial test based on the polymerase chain reaction for detecting *Mycobacterium tuberculosis* in respiratory specimens. Am J Respir Crit Care Med 1995;151:1872–1877.

PATIENT 36

A 62-year-old man with back pain, a paraspinal mass, and an abnormal chest radiograph

A 62-year-old man was admitted complaining of back pain, weight loss, and fever of 4 weeks duration. He denied a history of tuberculosis or contact with anyone known to have the disease.

Physical Examination: Temperature 101.5°F, pulse 88, respirations 14. General: chronically ill-appearing man. Chest: crackles in the upper lung fields bilaterally. Cardiac: normal. Abdomen: no organomegaly. Musculoskeletal: no spinal tenderness. Neurologic: normal motor strength.

Laboratory Findings: Hct 37%, WBC 14,500/μl. Electrolytes, liver functions tests: normal. Tuberculin skin test: 12 mm of induration at 48 hours. Chest radiograph: right upper lobe infiltrate. Chest CT scan (shown below): paraspinal soft tissue density at T_{12}-L_1 with extension into the anterior regions of adjacent vertebral bodies. Sputum acid-fast smear: positive.

Questions: What is the cause of the paraspinal mass? What therapeutic measures should be instituted?

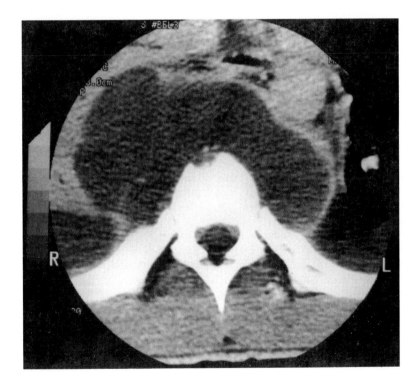

Diagnosis: Spinal tuberculosis (Pott's disease).

Discussion: Skeletal tuberculosis accounts for 9–10% of tuberculous infections in patients with the extrapulmonary form of the disease. Weight-bearing bones are the most commonly involved sites of infection because of their rich blood suppy that establishes a high oxygen environment conducive to the growth of *M. tuberculosis*. Skeletal tuberculosis, however, has been reported to occur in nearly any bone in the body. Up to 50% of patients with skeletal tuberculosis have the infection localized to the spine. The hips and knees (15–20% of cases) and shoulders, elbows, ankles, and wrists (15–20% of cases) account for most of the remaining cases. Most instances of skeletal tuberculosis occur as a result of reactivation disease from a foci seeded at the time of initial infection.

Skeletal tuberculosis is somewhat more common in older patients with tuberculosis; men and women have an equal incidence of the disease. Interestingly, a patient's age determines the likely location of infection in patients with Pott's disease. Young patients most often have involvement of the upper thoracic vertebrae, whereas adults experience disease in the lower thoracic and upper lumbar regions.

The findings of a paraspinal mass with destruction of an adjacent vertebral body in a patient with pulmonary tuberculosis is diagnostic of spinal tuberculosis. Diagnosis of Pott's disease is suspected when a patient presents with pulmonary tuberculosis and radiographic abnormalities of the spine detected by plain film, CT scanning, or MRI. Nearly 35% of patients with skeletal tuberculosis, however, have no evidence of pulmonary disease. Radiographic bony abnormalities include typical findings of osteomyelitis, including soft-tissue swelling, subchondral osteoporosis, cystic changes, and sclerosis. CT scans and MRI are significantly more sensitive than plain films for detecting the early presence of the disease. Although definitive diagnosis depends on the demonstration of acid-fast organisms on stained specimens (20–25% of cases) and positive cultures (80% of cases) of bone biopsy specimens, a presumptive diagnosis may be made if the characteristic clinical and radiographic findings are present in a patient with active pulmonary tuberculosis.

Controversy exists about the treatment of Pott's disease. Treatment issues that remain unclear include the optimal duration of chemotherapy and the role of spinal surgery. Although accumulating evidence supports the efficacy of short-course chemotherapy for extrapulmonary tuberculosis, these regimens have not been widely evaluated in this clinical setting. As a result, recent recommendations from the American Thoracic Society and the Centers for Disease Control and Prevention are that tuberculosis of the bones and joints be treated for at least 12 months, as opposed to the standard 6-month therapy for isolated pulmonary disease.

Regarding the role of spinal surgery in Pott's disease, general consensus exists that neurologically intact patients can be treated with antituberculous drug therapy alone. Nearly all of these patient will experience a microbiologic cure, although a residual kyphosis occurs in many patients. Several older studies report a kyphosis of more than 10° in 40% of patients treated with medical therapy alone. Most of these patients, however, had a favorable functional outcome as defined by the resumption of normal full activity. Other studies indicate that neurologically intact patients do not require immobilization of the spine in addition to antituberculous drug therapy.

If focal neurologic deficits or spinal instability are present, early surgical intervention may be beneficial. The range of possible procedures includes vertebrectomy with bone grafting, spinal stabilization with placement of rods, laminectomy, and extradural decompression of a paraspinal abscess. Many surgeons believe that simple debridement should be done only for diagnosis, and surgical intervention, if indicated at all, should be extensive and definitive to ensure the resolution of neurologic deficits and spinal instability. An additional indication for surgical intervention is a lack of response to medical therapy.

The present patient had no evidence of neurologic impairment or spinal instability. He was treated with antituberculous chemotherapy for 12 months without surgical intervention. He responded well to therapy, recovering full function and resuming his normal range of activities.

Clinical Pearls

1. Pott's disease should be suspected in patients with back pain, fever, and positive tuberculin tests, whether or not the chest radiograph suggests active disease.

2. Plain radiographs of the spine may not detect abnormalities in patients with early Pott's disease. CT scanning or MRI have greater sensitivity. Unless active pulmonary disease is diagnosed, patients in whom Pott's disease is suspected should undergo closed needle or open surgical biopsy of the vertebral lesions.

3. Patients with Pott's disease who have neurologic findings or spinal instability should undergo surgical intervention in addition to drug therapy. Patients with intact neurologic examinations have good response to chemotherapy alone.

REFERENCES

1. Janssens JP, Dehaller R. Spinal tuberculosis in a developed country: a review of 26 cases with special emphasis on abscesses and neurological complications. Clin Orthop 1990;257:67–78.
2. Jain R, Sawhney S, Berry M. Computed tomography of vertebral tuberculosis: patterns of bone destruction. Clin Radiol 1993;47:196–199.
3. Medical Research Council Working Party on Tuberculosis of the Spine. Twelfth report: controlled trial of short course regimens of chemotherapy in the ambulatory treatment of spinal tuberculosis. J Bone Joint Surg (Br) 1993;75:240–248.
4. Rezai AR, Lee M, Cooper PR, et al. Modern management of spinal tuberculosis. Neurosurgery 1995;36:87–98.

PATIENT 37

A 53-year-old man with a neck mass and an abnormal chest radiograph

A 53-year-old man with a history of asthma, intravenous drug abuse, and HIV infection presented with fever, cough, a left neck mass, and an abnormal chest radiograph. He had a history of tobacco use and admitted to actively using intravenous drugs. There was no history of previous tuberculosis or prior positive tuberculin skin test. The patient denied contact with anyone with known tuberculosis.

Physical Examination: Temperature 101.5°F, other vital signs normal. General: chronically ill-appearing man. Head: normal. Neck: fluctuant 2×3 cm left posterior neck mass. Chest: normal. Heart: normal heart sounds, without murmurs or rubs. Abdomen: normal. Extremities: normal. Neurologic: normal.

Laboratory Findings: Hct 42%, WBC 3,700/μl, electrolytes: normal. CD4+ cell count: 145/μl. Chest radiograph: shown below. Left neck mass aspirate: purulent material containing gram-positive cocci in clusters. A culture of the material yielded *Staphylococcus aureus*. Induced sputum sample: positive for acid-fast organisms.

Question: What relationships exist between the patient's history of HIV disease and drug abuse and the findings of a neck mass and abnormal chest radiograph?

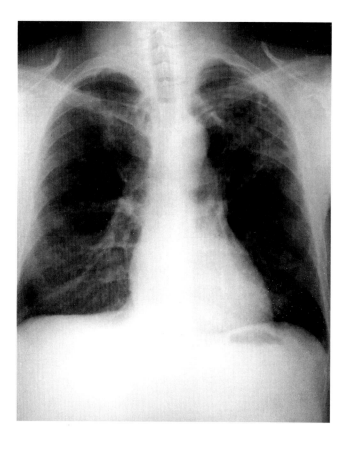

Diagnosis: Pulmonary tuberculosis in an HIV-infected patient. Neck abscess from injecting drugs into cervical veins.

Discussion: Pulmonary tuberculosis is a frequent complication of HIV infection, being now recognized as an AIDS-defining illness in the presence of HIV infection. In cities such as New York, where AIDS and tuberculosis are common, roughly one-half of patients with tuberculosis are HIV-infected. It appears clear that to a great extent HIV infection has fueled the current tuberculosis epidemic in the United States.

The two diseases, tuberculosis and HIV infection, are directly linked by the primary immune defect in AIDS, which is an impairment of cellular immunity caused by a depletion of CD4+ T-cells, and the dependence of the host on cellular immune defenses to control *M. tuberculosis*. Demographic features such as intravenous drug use and homelessness, frequent among patients with HIV infection in inner city settings, are also associated with higher rates of tuberculosis, further linking the two diseases. In areas where both tuberculosis and HIV infection are common, all patients with tuberculosis should be urged to undergo HIV testing.

A great deal of discussion regarding the clinical presentation of pulmonary tuberculosis in patients with AIDS has emphasized the atypical radiographic findings in this patient population. In actual fact, the radiographic manifestations of tuberculosis in AIDS patients are generally quite typical for tuberculosis if they are considered as representing primary disease. Indeed, patients with HIV infection have a high incidence of primary tuberculosis, which follows an accelerated progressive course. The radiographic manifestations of primary tuberculosis include isolated hilar or mediastinal lymphadenopathy, pleural effusions, and patchy lower lobe infiltrates representing tuberculous pneumonia, and a lower incidence of cavitary parenchymal disease. Normal chest radiographs in HIV-positive patients have also been reported in conjunction with positive sputum cultures; these patients should be treated for active pulmonary tuberculosis. Any of these findings in patients with HIV infection and a subacute symptom complex should raise the clinician's index of suspicion, and tuberculosis should be specifically ruled out.

Despite the relative frequency of tuberculosis in HIV-infected patients, investigators have noted frequent delays in the diagnosis of tuberculosis in this patient population. One study found delays in institution of therapy of at least 3 weeks from time of presentation in nearly 50% of consecutive HIV-positive patients with tuberculosis. These delays appear to result from a failure to consider tuberculosis in the differential diagnosis on admission and subsequent delays in obtaining appropriate sputum smears and cultures. In addition, physicians often demonstrate reluctance to begin antituberculous therapy empirically in patients who have clinical and radiographic signs of tuberculosis but negative sputum examinations.

The consequences of a delayed or missed diagnosis of tuberculosis in an HIV-infected patient can go far beyond the morbidity of the particular patient. Many nosocomial outbreaks of tuberculosis in HIV-infected patients have been reported in the literature, and each outbreak usually began with one unrecognized or untreated case. In Miami, 22 patients were reported to contract tuberculosis by contact with one inadequately treated person. Studies employing restriction fragment length polymorphism (RFLP analysis, also known as DNA fingerprinting) have proved conclusively that such outbreaks, such as one involving 18 patients in a New York City hospital, can be traced to an infectious source case.

In the present patient bilateral upper and lower lobe infiltrates were compatible with the diagnosis of primary pulmonary tuberculosis. An induced sputum sample demonstrated acid-fast organisms, and the patient was begun on antituberculous medication. His neck abscess, which was caused by direct injection of intravenous drugs into that area, was treated with antibacterial agents. Sputum cultures eventually grew *M. tuberculosis* sensitive to all antituberculous agents, and the patient received a 9-month course of antituberculous therapy with isoniazid and rifampin, in accordance with ATS and CDC guidelines at the time. Currently, it is considered acceptable to treat HIV-infected patients with pan-sensitive isolates for 6 months if they have a good clinical response.

Clinical Pearls

1. A high clinical index of suspicion is crucial to making a diagnosis of pulmonary tuberculosis in patients with AIDS.

2. Specific etiologic diagnoses should always be sought in AIDS patients admitted with abnormal chest radiographs to avoid missing a tuberculosis infection.

3. Radiographic manifestations of tuberculosis in patients with HIV infection often represent primary tuberculosis, and include adenopathy, middle and lower lobe infiltrates, and pleural effusions. Some patients with positive sputum cultures have normal chest radiographs.

4. Failure to diagnose and treat tuberculosis in hospitalized AIDS patients may lead to nosocomial outbreaks that will affect scores of patients.

REFERENCES

1. Pitchenik AE, Rubinson HA. The radiographic appearance of tuberculosis in patients with the acquired immunodeficiency syndrome (AIDS) and pre-AIDS. Am Rev Respir Dis 1985;131:393–396.
2. Kramer F, Modilevsky T, Waliany AR, et al. Delayed diagnosis of tuberculosis in patients with human immunodeficiency virus infection. Am J Med 1990;89:451–456.
3. Fischl M, Uttamchandani RB, Daikos G, et al. An outbreak of tuberculosis caused by multiple-drug-resistant tubercle bacilli among patients with HIV infection. Ann Intern Med 1992;117:177–183.
4. Edlin BR, Tokars J, Grieco M, et al. An outbreak of multidrug-resistant tuberculosis among hospitalized patients with the acquired immunodeficiency syndrome. N Engl J Med 1992;326:1514–1521.

PATIENT 38

A 26-year-old woman with a positive tuberculin test after BCG vaccination in childhood

A 26-year-old woman was referred for evaluation of a pre-employment tuberculin skin test that was reactive at 22 mm of induration. The patient felt well and had no previous medical history. She was a nurse who had recently emigrated from the Philippines. As a child she had received a BCG vaccination. To the best of her memory, her reaction to a tuberculin test was "always positive." She denied risk factors for HIV infection.

Physical Examination: Normal.

Laboratory Findings: Chest radiograph: Normal. HIV test: negative.

Question: Does the positive tuberculin reaction represent successful BCG vaccination or infection with tuberculosis?

Diagnosis: Tuberculosis infection.

Discussion: Although 3 billion individuals have been vaccinated with the bacillus of Calmette and Guérin (BCG) since its first use in 1921, controversy over the efficacy and appropriate use of the vaccine abounds.

BCG is a nonvirulent strain of the tubercle bacillus originally developed by repeatedly subculturing a strain obtained from an infected cow. Early techniques of vaccine production led to heterogeneity of strains used for vaccination. Recognition of this problem led to modern techniques and standards that maintain homogeneity within strains. Of the vaccines used today, 90% are produced from one of three parent strains, of which the Pasteur Institute strain is the international reference standard. Originally given by the oral route, today the vaccine is most commonly administered by intradermal injection, although percutaneous scarification may also be used. The intradermal route produces a pustule that heals within 3 months, producing a scar at the vaccination site.

Although BCG is considered one of the safest vaccines in use, adverse reactions due to injection of a live attenuated bacillus do occur. The most common serious complication is local suppurative lymphadenitis, which usually occurs within 5 months of inoculation at a rate of 2.5 per 100,000. As children under 1 year of age are particularly susceptible to this complication, they should receive only 0.05 ml of vaccine, one-half of the dose given to older children. Optimal treatment of this complication is unclear, as spontaneous resolution can occur; surgical drainage or removal of the nodes may be required, because antituberculous medications are generally ineffective. Osteomyelitis of the epiphysis of the long bones may occur within 2 years of vaccination at a rate of 0.1 per 100,000, although patients may present with this complication as much as 10 years later. Medical treatment with antituberculous agents is usually effective, although surgical intervention may be necessary. Disseminated BCG disease is a rare but usually fatal complication that is almost never seen in immunocompetent patients. Although this complication has been observed in patients with AIDS, BCG has not been demonstrated to be unsafe in HIV-infected patients without AIDS; conversely, efficacy in these patients has not been studied.

Efficacy of BCG in general remains uncertain, despite the large number of studies addressing this concern. The protection against tuberculosis in various prospective trials ranges from zero to 80%, and even a detrimental effect has been suggested. The largest controlled trial, begun in Madras, India in 1968 and involving over 250,000 individuals over 1 month of age, failed to demonstrate any protection against pulmonary tuberculosis. Explanations offered for the disparity of results include methodologic problems of trials and differences in potency between different strains. A recent meta-analysis that selected data from all known studies of the effectiveness of BCG vaccination found a reduction in the risk of tuberculosis of 50%. Age at vaccination did not affect efficacy, and protection against disseminated tuberculosis, tuberculous meningitis, and death from tuberculosis was higher than protection against pulmonary tuberculosis. Despite the uncertainty of efficacy, tuberculosis remains such a major public health problem worldwide that the World Health Organization continues to recommend vaccination for infants; the majority of countries in the world use BCG vaccination.

Effects of BCG vaccination on the tuberculin skin test are variable and depend on such factors as dose of vaccine, number of vaccinations, age of recipient, immune status, and interval between vaccination and tuberculin testing. Maximal response to tuberculin develops 12 weeks after inoculation and is rarely more than 15 mm. The response decreases with time, possibly starting as quickly as 18 months later. As few as 5% of children may react to tuberculin 5 years after vaccination. Therefore, although BCG vaccination renders interpretation of the tuberculin test problematic, it is safe to say that the more remote the vaccination, and the larger the induration, the greater the likelihood that a positive response represents tuberculosis infection. BCG vaccination in early childhood should not affect the interpretation of a tuberculin test in an adult.

The combination of uncertain efficacy, potential effects on future tuberculin testing, and the low risk of tuberculosis in the general population greatly limits the usefulness of the vaccine in the United States. Therefore it is currently recommended for use only in children with negative skin tests who cannot be removed from exposure to: (1) patients with infectious tuberculosis who remain untreated or ineffectively treated, if the child cannot be given long-term preventive therapy, or (2) infectious patients with multidrug-resistant tuberculosis. It is also recommended for use in tuberculin-negative children in populations in which the rate of new infection exceeds 1% per year and for whom usual surveillance and treatment programs are not feasible.

The tuberculin skin test in the current patient was interpreted as positive for tuberculosis infection due the remoteness of vaccination. She was treated with isoniazid preventive therapy for 6 months in accordance with current guidelines.

Clinical Pearls

1. Despite the vast experience with BCG vaccination, its efficacy remains unclear. A meta-analysis of available evidence suggests it significantly reduces the risk of tuberculosis by about 50%.

2. BCG vaccine may provide better protection against disseminated tuberculosis, tuberculous meningitis, and death from tuberculosis than against pulmonary tuberculosis.

3. Because BCG is a live attenuated mycobacterium, disease from the organism, such as local lymphadenitis, osteomyelitis, and fatal dissemination, may rarely occur.

4. The reaction to tuberculin skin testing after BCG vaccination is variable and wanes with time; in an adult vaccinated during childhood, a positive tuberculin skin test is most likely due to tuberculosis infection.

5. Although BCG may play an important role in tuberculosis control in developing countries where the risk of tuberculosis is high, and it is recommended for use in children worldwide, its usefulness in the United States is restricted to isolated, well-defined situations.

REFERENCES

1. World Health Organization. Vaccination against tuberculosis. WHO/Technical Report Series 651, 1980.
2. Tripathy SP. Fifteen-year follow-up of the Indian BCG prevention trial. Bull Int Union Tuberc 1987;62:69–72.
3. Centers for Disease Control. Use of BCG vaccines in the control of tuberculosis: a joint statement by the ACIP and the Advisory Committee for Elimination of Tuberculosis. MMWR 1988;37:663–664, 669–675.
4. Menzies R, Vissandjee B. Effect of bacille Calmette-Guérin vaccination on tuberculin reactivity. Am Rev Respir Dis 1992;145:621–625.
5. Colditz GA, Brewer TF, Berkey CS, et al. Efficacy of BCG vaccine in the prevention of tuberculosis: meta-analysis of the published literature. JAMA 1994;271:698–702.

PATIENT 39

A 4-year-old boy with an enlarged cardiac silhouette

A 4-year-old boy from Santo Domingo was brought to the pediatric clinic by his mother because of a 1-week history of nonproductive cough, decreased activity, weight loss, fever, and poor appetite. The child had no significant medical history, and had experienced normal growth and development to date. The mother did not know if the boy had received BCG vaccination in Santo Domingo. The family had immigrated to the United States 8 months earlier. The mother did not know of any exposure to tuberculosis, and no other family members were ill.

Physical Examination: Temperature 100.3°F, pulse 120, respirations 32, blood pressure 108/50, without pulsus paradoxus. Head: normal. Lungs: decreased breath sounds and dullness at left base, otherwise clear. Heart: point of maximal impulse diffuse and laterally displaced, S_1 and S_2 normal, friction rub present. Abdomen: normal.

Laboratory Findings: Hct 30%, WBC 5,900/µl, platelets 500,000/µl. Electrolytes, renal indices, liver function tests: normal. Chest radiograph: enlarged cardiac silhoutte. Chest CT (shown below): enlarged cardiac silhouette, splayed carina, bilateral hilar adenopathy, left lower lobe infiltrate, and left pleural effusion. EKG: normal voltage, axis 60°, sinus tachycardia. Echocardiogram: Large posterior pericardial effusion, thickened "shaggy"-appearing pericardium, no evidence of tamponade, normal myocardial contractility. Tuberculin skin test: 15 mm of induration. Gastric aspirates: 3 samples negative for acid-fast bacilli.

Question: What is the proper management of pericarditis in this patient?

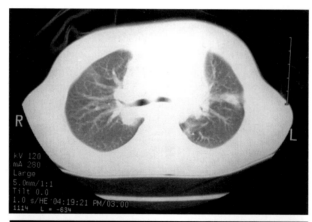

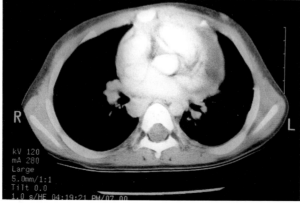

Diagnosis: Tuberculous pericarditis.

Discussion: Pericarditis is an unusual manifestation of tuberculosis, making up a small fraction of all patients with extrapulmonary disease. Less than 10% of all instances of acute pericarditis are due to tuberculosis, except in some underdeveloped countries where tuberculosis is overwhelmingly the most common cause of pericardial disease.

Tuberculous pericarditis typically evolves from a subclinical fibrinous stage through an effusive stage during which fluid accumulates in the pericardial sac. Over several days the fluid becomes increasingly turbid as the pericardium thickens and becomes coated with a fibrinous exudate, which lends a shaggy appearance to the pericardial surface. Initially, the predominant inflammatory cell is the polymorphonuclear cell, which in the next few days gives way to a lymphocytic predominance. This is analogous to changes in the cellular composition of the fluid observed in tuberculous pleurisy. Granuloma formation continues to cause pericardial thickening as the effusion begins to resolve. Finally the pericardium becomes fibrotic as the granulomatous inflammation subsides, and constrictive pericarditis may ensue as the fibrous tissue contracts.

Patients with tuberculous pericarditis are most commonly young adults who typically present with fever, cough, dyspnea, and chest pain; orthopnea, jugular venous distention, hepatic congestion, and pedal edema are less common, but their presence in a patient with tuberculosis should alert the clinician to the potential of pericardial involvement. Less than one-third of patients will present with overt cardiac tamponade. Most patients will have a concomitant left-sided pleural effusion, but only one-third will have an accompanying pulmonary parenchymal infiltrate.

Confirming tuberculosis as the cause of the pericardial disease may be difficult. All patients should have the pericardial fluid examined, but acid-fast bacilli are rarely found and standard cultures may grow *M. tuberculosis* in only 25%–50% of patients. Inoculation of double-strength Kirchner medium at the bedside may increase the yield of fluid culture to 60–75%. Pericardial biopsy provides a rapid diagnosis, revealing typical granulomatous inflammation in up to three-quarters of patients, although yields as low as 29% have been reported. Tuberculin skin tests are almost always positive in immunocompetent hosts, although in one series of children with tuberculous pericarditis, 26% did not react to tuberculin. Several authors have found elevated levels of adenosine deaminase activity in pericardial fluid to be indicative of tuberculosis (as is also true when found in pleural fluid), and others have advocated using the polymerase chain reaction technique on pericardial fluid to detect *M. tuberculosis*.

Routine chest radiographs revealing an enlarged cardiac silhouette are nonspecific for the diagnosis of tuberculous pericarditis, although findings typical of pulmonary tuberculosis are helpful when present. Echocardiography should be performed in all patients to confirm noninvasively the presence of pericardial fluid and evaluate possible tamponade. This technique can detect pericardial thickening in about one-half of patients, allowing distinction from restrictive pericarditis. When present, the appearance of a "shaggy" pericardium is particularly suggestive of tuberculous pericarditis. CT and MRI scans are also sensitive ways of demonstrating thickened pericardium.

Although the advent of antituberculous chemotherapy has helped in reducing the mortality of tuberculous pericarditis from rates as high as 80%, the optimal role of pericardial drainage procedures and use of steroids in further minimizing mortality has only recently begun to emerge. Clearly, all patients should receive antituberculous chemotherapy, following the recommendations for treatment of pulmonary tuberculosis. Systemic corticosteroids have been shown to reduce mortality from tuberculous pericarditis, but do not seem to decrease later development of constrictive pericarditis or the need for eventual pericardiectomy. Doses in the range of 40–80 mg of prednisone or its equivalent are usually given in adults, tapering the dose over 2–3 months. It should be remembered that rifampin increases the rate of metabolism of steroids by induction of hepatic enzymes, so the dose may need to be increased.

Pericardiocentesis with catheter drainage seems a reasonable initial approach in most patients, and can be life-saving in patients with tamponade, although the majority in this group will require subsequent open drainage with a pericardial window or a pericardiectomy. The question of routine early pericardiectomy versus reservation of the procedure for patients who do not improve on medical therapy remains controversial, although its utility when constrictive pericarditis is present appears certain. Recent series combining antituberculous therapy, steroids, and surgical intervention in at least some selected patients report mortalities of zero to 14%.

Regarding the current patient, contact investigation of household members found that the mother and younger brother both had positive tuberculin tests and normal chest radiographs, while the father was tuberculin negative. The patient was given daily isoniazid 175 mg (10 mg/kg), rifampin 175 mg (10 mg/kg), pyrazinamide 500 mg (30 mg/kg), ethambutol 300 mg (15 mg/kg), and prednisone 30 mg. On the second hospital day a subxiphoid pericardiocentesis was performed, with pericardial biopsy and placement of a drain. The fluid was exudative, with protein of 5.1 g/L and a cell count of 8,200/μl, with lymphocytes predominating. Stain of the fluid was negative for acid-fast bacilli. Histologic examination of the biopsy specimen revealed necrotizing granulomata that stained negative for acid-fast bacilli. The patient was asymptomatic with resolution of the pericardial effusion after 2 months of therapy and remained well throughout the remainder of the therapeutic course.

Clinical Pearls

1. Tuberculous peridcarditis may have an acute presentation, mimicking bacterial pericarditis, or a subacute or chronic presentation. The key to diagnosis is demonstration of granuloma in the pericardium or recovery of organisms from pericardial fluid.

2. Recent published series indicate that outcome is better if the pericardial space is drained. This procedure markedly decreases the incidence of constrictive pericarditis.

3. The use of steroids is associated with improved outcome, although clinical benefit is observed most in patients whose pericardial space is not drained. If steroids are used, there should be little or no chance that the patient has multidrug-resistant tuberculosis.

REFERENCES

1. Strang JI, Gibson DG, Mitchison DA, et al. Controlled clinical trial of complete open surgical drainage and of prednisolone in treatment of tuberculous pericardial effusion in Transkei. Lancet 1988;2:759–764.
2. Chandraratna PA. Echocardiography and doppler ultrasound in the evaluation of pericardial disease. Circulation 1991; 84(Suppl 3):1103–1110.
3. Zahn EM, Houde C, Benson L, Freedom RM. Percutaneous pericardial catheter drainage in childhood. Am J Cardiol 1992;70:681–688.
4. Hugo-Hamman CT, Scher H, DeMoor MM. Tuberculous pericarditis in children: a review of 44 cases. Pediatr Infect Dis J 1994;13:13–18.

PATIENT 40

A 62-year-old man with back pain and a pleural effusion

A 62-year-old man presented with dyspnea and a left flank mass. The patient immigrated to the United States 8 years earlier from Cameroon where he had been treated for malaria. In addition, there was a history of a "lung tumor" for which he had been operated on several years earlier. His physicians had noted an enlarged liver that had persisted since his malarial illness.

Physical Examination: Temperature 102°F, other vital signs normal. General: comfortable. Head: normal. Chest: diminished breath sounds throughout left lung field, right lung field normal. Cardiac: normal heart sounds without murmurs, gallops, or rubs. Abdomen: distended, hepatomegaly, no fluid waves. Extremities: normal. Neurologic: normal.

Laboratory Findings: Hct 36%, WBC 7,000/μl. Electrolytes: normal. Chest radiograph (shown below): large left pleural effusion and surgical clips in the right mid-lung field. Pleural fluid: milky appearance, pH 7.42, protein 5.6 gm/dL, LDH 4,000 IU/L, leukocytes 944/μl with 64% lymphocytes, cholesterol 133 mg/dl, triglycerides 167 mg/dl, acid-fast stain positive for acid-fast organisms. Tuberculin test: positive with 15 mm induration.

Questions: How would this effusion be described? What is its pathogenesis?

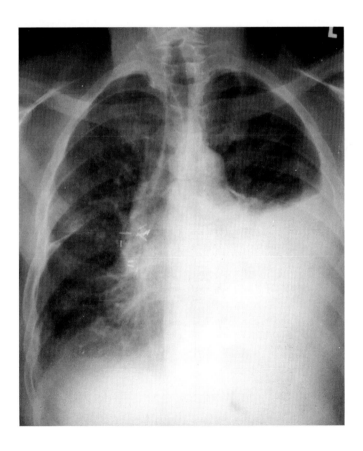

Diagnosis: Tuberculous pleurisy with a chylous effusion.

Discussion: Tuberculous pleural effusions are a common manifestation of tuberculosis that occur in up to 10% of patients. Although generally considered to occur in patients with primary disease, recent observations indicate that tuberculous pleurisy may also occur in patients with reactivated pulmonary tuberculosis in older age groups. Consequently, tuberculosis should be considered in elderly patients who present with pulmonary infiltrates and pleural effusions, especially when those patients reside in nursing homes where mini-epidemics of tuberculosis can occur.

As a manifestation of primary disease, tuberculous pleurisy is properly classified as an extrapulmonary form of tuberculosis. Patients present with varied manifestations that range from a subacute febrile illness to a syndrome that may mimic acute bacterial pneumonia or pulmonary thromboembolic disease. This varied presentation may mislead the clinician to consider alternative diagnoses. Furthermore, patients may "respond" to inappropriate therapy or simple observation because a large proportion of cases resolve in the absence of antituberculous chemotherapy. Approximately two-thirds of patients left untreated will progress to active pulmonary tuberculosis within the following 2–3 years.

Thoracentesis represents the cornerstone for considering the diagnosis of tuberculous pleurisy. Detection of exudative pleural fluid with a lymphocyte predominance in a patient with an otherwise unexplained pleural effusion should raise clinical suspicion. The likelihood of tuberculous pleurisy is especially high in this setting if the patient is younger than 35 years of age. In patients with primary disease, the concentration of tubercle bacilli in the pleural space is low, so culture and direct examination of pleural fluid are positive in only 20% of patients. In addition, tuberculin skin tests are often negative in this disease at the time of clinical presentation.

Pleural biopsy is often required to establish the diagnosis of tuberculous pleurisy. Demonstration of granulomata on pleural specimens can establish a presumptive diagnosis that allows early initiation of antituberculous therapy. Combining culture and histopathologic results of thoracentesis and pleural tissue specimens can result in an established diagnosis in more than 90% of patients. In some instances, chemotherapy may be indicated in the presence of an unexplained lymphocyte-predominant exudative effusion in a patient with a positive tuberculin test, pending confirmation of the diagnosis, even if a pleural biopsy specimen fails to demonstrate granulomata. In this setting, a malignant pleural effusion must be excluded because this condition can generate a similar pleural fluid profile.

The presence of milky-appearing pleural fluid is an unusual but described manifestation of tuberculous pleurisy that may be attributed to a chylous or a pseudochylous effusion. Chylous effusions are defined by a pleural fluid triglyceride concentration above 110 mg/dl and result from mechanical disruption or blockage of the thoracic duct. The vast majority of such effusions are related to intrathoracic malignancies (usually lymphomas) with mediastinal involvement. Tuberculosis is one of the rare "miscellaneous" causes of chylous effusions in a category that includes filariasis, amyloidosis, sarcoidosis, and lymphangioleiomyomatosis. These etiologies account for 10% of all chylous effusions. Pseudochylous effusions have low triglyceride concentrations but high cholesterol contents. These effusions occur in chronic tuberculous pleurisy when the pleural fluid fails to resolve. The source of cholesterol is breakdown of intrapleural cells.

Nearly all patients with tuberculous pleural effusions can be treated successfully with antituberculous chemotherapy. Drainage of the pleural space is necessary only in cases of tuberculous empyema in which frank pus is present. In tuberculous chylothorax, the thoracic duct obstruction is presumably due to an enlarged lymph node, which should shrink with drug therapy.

The present patient's lymphocyte-predominant exudative pleural effusion with a high triglyceride content and positive acid-fast organisms was consistent with tuberculous chylous effusion. The patient was treated initially with isoniazid, rifampin, ethambutol, and pyrazinamide, and gradually improved with resolution of the pleural effusion. Pleural fluid cultures were positive for drug-sensitive *M. tuberculosis*.

Clinical Pearls

1. Pleural effusions can occur in both primary and reactivation tuberculosis, although the former scenario is more common.

2. A high index of suspicion, triggered by the finding of a lymphocyte-predominant exudative effusion, is required to make the diagnosis of tuberculous pleurisy, as this entity has many mimics.

3. Although unusual, it is possible for tuberculosis to cause a chylous effusion, and this diagnosis should be entertained particularly in patients with chylous effusions not explainable by tumors or trauma.

REFERENCES

1. Vennera M, Morena R, Cot J, et al. Chylothorax and tuberculosis. Thorax 1983;38:694–695.
2. Valentine VG, Raffin TA. The management of chylothorax. Chest 1992;102:586–591.
3. Ferguson MK. Thoracoscopy for empyema, bronchopleural fistula, and chylothorax. Ann Thorac Surg 1993;56:644–645.
4. Paes ML, Powell H. Chylothorax: an update. Br J Hosp Med 1994;51:482–490.

PATIENT 41

A 27-year-old man with a positive tuberculin skin test and a history of exposure to multidrug-resistant tuberculosis

A 27-year-old man presented for evaluation of a positive tuberculin skin test. The patient reported that his roommate had died 6 months earlier of tuberculosis. The patient felt well and denied fevers, chills, sweats, cough, or weight loss. His previous health had been good, although he did occasionally use illicit intravenous drugs. The patient stated that a tuberculin skin test performed 1 year earlier had been negative.

Physical Examination: Vital signs: normal. General: comfortable. The remainder of the physical examination was entirely normal.

Laboratorory Findings: CBC, electrolytes, liver function tests: normal. Tuberculin skin test: 12 mm of induration at 48 hours. HIV test: negative. Chest radiograph: normal. Review of records of the department of health revealed that the isolate recovered from the patient's roommate was resistant to isoniazid and rifampin.

Question: What therapy, if any, should be prescribed for the management of the positive tuberculin skin test?

Diagnosis: Tuberculosis infection likely due to multidrug-resistant tuberculosis (MDR-TB).

Discussion: The ongoing spread of multidrug-resistant (MDR) tuberculosis presents an increasingly important challenge in the management of patients with positive tuberculin skin tests. Guidelines based on empiric data exist for recommending preventive therapy for patients with positive tuberculin skin tests who have been exposed to drug-sensitive organisms. Unfortunately, no such data support the recommendations for managing patients with positive skin tests who have been exposed to individuals with MDR infections. Preventive therapy is largely based on expert consensus.

The Centers for Disease Control and Prevention (CDC) recommends that clinicians estimate the likelihood of infection with MDR organisms before instituting preventive therapy in any patient with a positive tuberculin skin test. This estimate is based on the infectiousness of the source case, the closeness and intensity of the MDR exposure, and the contact's risk of exposure to drug-susceptible tuberculosis. Finally, the CDC recommends making an assessment of the likelihood that a person infected with MDR tuberculosis will develop active disease. For patients with a strong likelihood of having been infected with MDR strains and who are at high risk for developing active disease, the CDC suggests that a preventive regimen consisting of at least two antituberculosis drugs be strongly considered. For contacts without HIV infection and not otherwise at high risk for developing active disease, the CDC suggests two options: either no preventive therapy at all, with extremely close clinical follow-up, or institution of multidrug preventive therapy. The CDC suggests regimens of either pyrazinamide and ethambutol (at doses used to treat active disease) daily for 6–12 months, or a combination of a quinolone (ciprofloxacin or ofloxacin) and pyrazinamide daily for 6–12 months. Few toxicity data for long-term administration of quinolones are available.

A provocative study using the Delphi technique to survey the attitudes and recommendations of expert physicians regarding treatment of MDR contacts has recently been published and contains conclusions similar to those of the CDC. Physicians were given a set of clinical scenarios and asked to choose from several potential chemoprophylactic regimens. The potential prophylactic regimens were either single-agent treatment with isoniazid or two-drug regimens consisting of pyrazinamide in combination with a quinolone, ethambutol, or streptomycin. The study demonstrated that the panel of experts did not consider any of the proposed options to be extremely appropriate for any proposed scenario, but regimens consisting of pyrazinamide and a quinolone, for a duration of 4 months, were most often believed to be appropriate for individuals very likely to have been infected with MDR tuberculosis who are at high risk for developing active disease.

The lack of regimens of proven efficacy in prevention of MDR tuberculosis for infected persons has prompted some to recommend vaccination with BCG for persons at high risk for contact with MDR cases. This would include certain health care workers in areas where MDR tuberculosis is prevalent. This recommendation cannot be considered a strong one, however, for two reasons. First, it remains unclear that BCG vaccination actually prevents tuberculosis. Second, patients treated with BCG convert their skin tests to positive, thereby obviating the value of this screening examination.

Because there exist *no* regimens of proven efficacy for preventing the occurrence of active disease in patients exposed to MDR strains, all exposed patients, whether placed on preventive regimens with zero, one, or two drugs, must be closely monitored. Follow-up with clinical and radiographic evaluations at 3–6-month intervals for 2 years following skin test conversion may be reasonable, particularly if the no therapy option is chosen.

The patient presented had clear indications for preventive therapy: he was young, a new skin test converter, a close contact of a recent case, and in a high-risk group for the development of AIDS from illicit drug abuse, although he was presently free of HIV infection. Because he was exposed to a patient with an MDR strain, he was treated for 4 months with a regimen containing pyrazinamide and a quinolone. He has not developed active disease during 2 years of follow-up.

Clinical Pearls

1. When a patient with a positive tuberculin skin test gives a history of exposure to a case of MDR tuberculosis, every effort must be made to assess the likelihood that the source truly has MDR disease, the intensity of the exposure, and the likelihood that the exposed patient will develop active disease.

2. If the circumstances favor preventive therapy in a patient exposed to MDR tuberculosis, the combination of pyrazinamide and a quinolone, for at least 4 months, may be appropriate. If the contact was exposed to a strain resistant to more than isoniazid and rifampin, the preventive regimen must be designed on the basis of drug susceptibility testing results.

3. No efficacy data are available for any preventive regimen for MDR tuberculosis, so physicians must follow patients extremely closely when they are being so treated.

REFERENCES

1. Gorzynski EA, Gutman SI, Allen W. Comparative antimycobacterial activities of difloxacin, temafloxacin, enoxacin, pefloxacin, reference quinolones, and a new macrolide, clarithromycin. Antimicrob Agents Chemother 1989;33:591–592.
2. Centers for Disease Control. Management of persons exposed to multidrug-resistant tuberculosis. MMWR 1992;41(No. RR-11):61–71.
3. Cohn DL, Iseman MD. Treatment and prevention of multidrug-resistant tuberculosis. Res Microbiol 1993;144:150–153.
4. Horn DL, Hewitt D, Alfalla C, et al. Limited tolerance of ofloxacin and pyrazinamide prophylaxis against tuberculosis. N Engl J Med 1994;330:1241.
5. Passanante MR, Gallagher CT, Reichman LB. Preventive therapy for contacts of multidrug-resistant tuberculosis: a Delphi survey. Chest 1994;106:431–434.

PATIENT 42

A 22-year-old postpartum woman with a productive cough and an abnormal chest radiograph

A 22-year-old woman who did not receive prenatal care presented to the hospital in active labor. She delivered a healthy infant via spontaneous vaginal birth. Post-partum, the woman gave a history of a cough productive of yellow sputum for 2–3 weeks before delivery. There was no other significant past medical history.

Physical Examination: Temperature 100.5°F, pulse 88, respirations 20, blood pressure 110/70. General: comfortable. HEENT: normal. Chest: scattered crackles bilaterally. Abdomen: post-partum. Extremities: normal. Neurologic: normal.

Laboratory Findings: Hct 28%, WBC 5,500/µl. Electrolytes and liver function tests: normal. Chest radiograph: right upper lung zone infiltrates, right-sided volume loss, and calcified hilar lymph nodes. Sputum smears: positive for acid-fast bacilli.

Question: What diagnostic and therapeutic measures, if any, should be taken regarding the newborn baby?

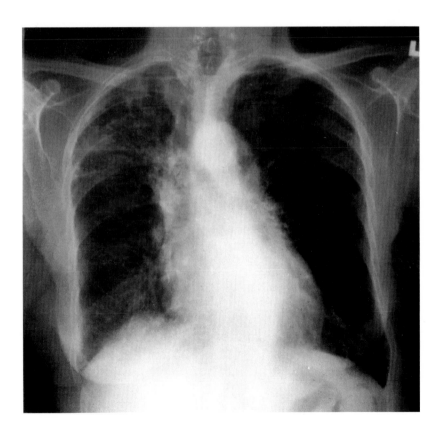

Diagnosis: Active pulmonary tuberculosis in a mother with a new infant.

Discussion: In considering the management of a mother with active tuberculosis and her newborn infant, different clinical approaches are required for the mother and child. As for the mother, no alterations of standard treatment regimens are required if she has drug-susceptible disease. Antituberculous drugs do not reach sufficient levels in mother's milk to prevent breast feeding. As for the infant, several issues require careful consideration. Foremost, it is critically important to establish whether the infant already has tuberculosis.

Tuberculosis among infants is relatively rare, although acquisition of infection can occur by two mechanisms. There can be transmission of mycobacteria in utero (true congenital tuberculosis) or airborne transmission from the mother after birth. True congenital tuberculosis is apparently extremely rare. From 1952 until 1980, only 24 cases of congenital tuberculosis were reported in the literature, and only an additional 29 cases have been reported since 1980. In utero transmission may occur directly through the placental circulation or possibly by aspiration of contaminated amniotic fluid. Accordingly, the focus of infection in the infant may be in the lungs, liver, or gastrointestinal tract.

The diagnosis of congenital tuberculosis is suggested by failure to thrive or the presence of jaundice. The infant's chest radiograph is often, but not always, abnormal. Tuberculin skin tests very early in life are usually negative even in the presence of active disease. Further complicating diagnosis, not all instances of congenital tuberculosis occurs in infants with mothers who have active disease. Determination that infantile tuberculosis is congenital in etiology by the criteria proposed in 1935 by Bietzke requires the presence of proven tuberculous lesions in the infant and one of the following: (1) lesions present soon after birth; (2) a primary hepatic complex; or (3) the exclusion of postnatal transmission by the separation of the infant at birth from the mother and other sources of infection. Recently proposed criteria for infants with proven tuberculosis require at least one of the following: (1) lesions in the first week of life; (2) a primary hepatic complex or caseating hepatic granulomas; (3) tuberculous infection of the placenta or genital tract; or (4) exclusion of the possibility of postnatal transmission.

Neonatally acquired tuberculosis due to airborne transmission presents most often with an abnormal chest radiograph. The diagnosis is generally established by positive endotracheal or gastric aspirates.

Treatment of neonatal tuberculosis is problematic because the disease is associated with substantial mortality, even when appropriate therapy is given. Also, adverse effects of medications are difficult to assess in infants. For these reasons, most authorities recommend treatment with isoniazid, rifampin, and pyrazinamide, with streptomycin or ethambutol added in serious infections. Unfortunately, most instances of neonatal tuberculosis are serious in nature. Streptomycin is often preferred over ethambutol because of the difficulty of monitoring for optic neuritis related to ethambutol toxicity in children. Eye problems are quite unusual, however, at the typically used ethambutol doses of 15 mg/kg.

If an infant born to a mother with active tuberculosis proves not to have tuberculosis, the child should be placed on isoniazid for at least 3 months or until the mother has been culture negative for 3 months, whichever occurs last. If a tuberculin skin test done at that time is negative, isoniazid can be stopped; if the infant is tuberculin positive, a full course of preventive therapy should be given. If there is a question of the compliance of the mother with antituberculous therapy, or if there is proven or suspected multidrug-resistant tuberculosis in the mother, strong consideration should be given to separating the infant from the mother until the mother is rendered noninfectious. This may appear to be a particularly harsh measure, but considering the mortality of neonatal tuberculosis, it seems justified. Finally, if the infant cannot be adequately protected by any of the above measures, it may be prudent to consider vaccination with BCG as a last resort, although the efficacy of this strategy is unknown.

The mother presented above proved to have drug-susceptible tuberculosis and complied with a course of standard drugs. Her infant was disease free and later proved to be tuberculin negative. The infant was given isoniazid for 3 months, after which the mother's sputum was smear and culture negative.

Clinical Pearls

1. Neonatal tuberculosis, either congenital or acquired, is an uncommon but potentially devastating disease. A careful evaluation of an infant born to a mother with tuberculosis should be initiated.

2. The most effective strategy to protect an infant from neonatally acquired tuberculosis is to assure that the mother is treated with an effective antituberculous regimen.

3. If the mother has active tuberculosis, vaccination with BCG may be appropriate for an infant without active disease if other preventive measures appear likely to be unsuccessful.

REFERENCES

1. Beitzke H. Uber die angeborene tuberkuloese infektion. Ergeb Gesamten Tuberkuloseforsch 1935;7:1.
2. Stansberry SD. Tuberculosis in infants and children. J Thorac Imag 1990;5:17–27.
3. Machin GA, Honore LH, Fanning EA, Molesky M. Perinatally acquired neonatal tuberculosis: report of two cases. Pediatr Pathol 1992;12:707–715.
4. Foo AL, Tan KK, Chay OM. Congenital tuberculosis. Tuberc Lung Dis 1993;74:59–61.
5. Cantwell MF, Shehab Z, Costello AM, et al. Brief report: congenital tuberculosis. N Engl J Med 1994;330:1051–1054.

PATIENT 43

A 29-year-old man with a supraclavicular mass that developed during antituberculous drug therapy

A 29-year-old homeless alcoholic man presented with a right supraclavicular mass. Two months earlier, he had begun daily directly observed therapy with isoniazid, rifampin, pyrazinamide, and ethambutol for a diagnosis of tuberculous pleurisy. His chest radiograph at that time was normal except for a moderate-sized pleural effusion. Culture of a pleural biopsy specimen grew *M. tuberculosis* that was susceptible to all tested drugs. The patient presently felt well. He had smoked 1 pack of cigarettes per day for 15 years and denied risk factors for HIV disease.

Physical Examination: Vital signs: normal. General: well-appearing man. Neck: 2x2 cm firm, slightly mobile nontender right supraclavicular node. Chest: normal. Cardiac: normal heart sounds. Abdomen: no organomegaly.

Laboratory Findings: CBC, electrolytes, liver function tests: normal. HIV test: negative. Chest radiograph (shown below): resolution of the previous pleural effusion. Chest CT (shown below): large subcarinal, paratracheal, and cervical lymph nodes with low density centers. Core aspirate of supraclavicular mass: granulomatous inflammation; aspirate Gram stain and acid-fast smear: negative; routine and acid-fast cultures: negative. Antituberculous serum drug levels: all in therapeutic range.

Question: What is the most likely cause of this patient's adenopathy?

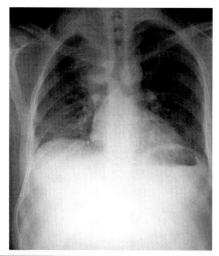

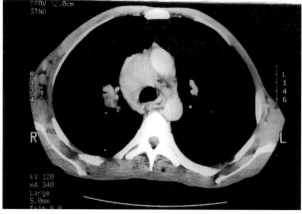

Diagnosis: Paradoxical enlargement of lymph nodes following institution of antituberculous chemotherapy.

Discussion: Nearly all patients with tuberculosis due to drug-susceptible strains experience an excellent response to therapy if they take their medications. Occasional patients, however, may develop new lesions or apparent progression of their disease while on therapy. Such occurrences may be due to one of several possibilities: (1) drug-resistant organisms, (2) poor drug compliance, (3) the new lesions represent nontuberculous disease, (4) poor drug absorption, and (5) a paradoxical response to otherwise effective therapy. Drug susceptibility studies and directly observed therapy should eliminate the first two of these concerns in almost all patients. Whenever possible, the new lesions should be aspirated or biopsied to rule out the third possibility of nontuberculous disease. The two remaining possibilities merit further consideration.

As for the possibility of poor drug absorption, all of the orally administered first-line agents—isoniazid, rifampin, pyrazinamide, and ethambutol—are well absorbed in the gastrointestinal tract in most patients. Patients with AIDS, however, may have subtherapeutic serum drug levels because of malaborption of antituberculous medications due to AIDS-related enteropathy. It seems likely that other causes of malabsorption would likewise interfere with tuberculosis therapy. Serum drug levels, therefore, should be measured in patients who take their medications and have a known or suspected malabsorption syndrome when tuberculosis does not appear to be responding to therapy.

If infection with drug-resistant organisms, noncompliance with therapy, malabsorption, and nontuberculous disease have all been satisfactorily ruled out, a paradoxical response to treatment is probably the cause of the new lesions. In this condition, tissue sites of granulomatous inflammation enlarge, becoming clinically apparent or more apparent if initial abnormalities were present at the onset of antituberculous therapy. Paradoxical responses occur most commonly in lymph nodes, brain, and lung. The pathogenesis of this response is uncertain. Biopsy specimens from tissues demonstrating a paradoxical response show granulomatous inflammation frequently with acid-fast organisms present, but tissue cultures are usually sterile. These findings suggest that the paradoxical response is a hypersensitivity reaction to the release of tuberculous antigens.

Although the literature suggests that intrathoracic lymph node enlargement occurring during a course of appropriate therapy is not a rare event, many clinicians are unaware of this phenomenon. This unawareness may occur because serial chest radiographs that may detect paradoxical intrathoracic reactions are not performed, and the transient and asymptomatic nature of extrathoracic lymph enlargement may not cause them to be reported to physicians. Paradoxical responses in the brain, however, are less likely to be subclinical and have a tendency to present as symptomatic intracranial tuberculomas. A recent review of the literature found 26 cases of intracranial tuberculomas that developed during chemotherapy, with the presentations almost equally divided between focal neurologic abnormalities and seizures. Approximately half the patients had multiple tuberculomas demonstrated on CT scan. The brain lesions occurred after a mean of 2 months' duration of treatment.

Most patients with extracranial paradoxical reactions do not require adjustments in their antituberculous drug therapy because they usually respond to continued treatment. Patients with intracranial lesions and evidence of increased intracranial pressure, however, benefit from the addition of corticosteroids to rapidly relieve their neurologic symptoms. If the clinical picture is unclear, or if drug susceptibility testing is unavailable, two additional drugs should be added to the regimen while the patient is being further evaluated.

The present patient was considered to have a paradoxical reaction on the basis of the histopathologic evidence of granulomatous inflammation. He was continued on his antituberculous regimen and the lymphadenopathy resolved after several more months of therapy.

Clinical Pearls

1. Patients who develop apparent progression of tuberculosis while receiving appropriate chemotherapy may not be absorbing medications from the gastrointestinal tract; this problem may be of particular concern in patients with AIDS.

2. Serum levels of antituberculous agents should be measured in patients suspected of malabsorption if the tuberculosis does not appear to be responding to therapy. Higher drug doses may be required in some patients to achieve adequate serum drug concentrations.

3. Paradoxical responses to adequate chemotherapy may occur in tuberculosis, manifested by new or enlarging lesions in lymph nodes, brain, or lung.

4. Paradoxical responses may be caused by a hypersensitivity reaction to tuberculosis and do not mandate a change in therapy. Corticosteroids should be added, however, in patients with increased intracranial pressure caused by tuberculomas.

REFERENCES

1. Teoh R, Humphries MJ, O'Mahoney G. Symptomatic intracranial tuberculoma developing during treatment of tuberculosis: a report of 10 patients and review of the literature. Q J Med 1987;63:449–460.
2. Berning SE, Huitt GA, Iseman MD, Peloquin CA. Malabsorption of antituberculous medications by a patient with AIDS. N Engl J Med 1992;327:1817–1818.
3. Carter EJ, Mates M. Sudden enlargement of a deep cervical lymph node during and after treatment for pulmonary tuberculosis. Chest 1994;106:1896–1898.
4. Silman JB, Peters JI, Levine SM, Jenkinson SG. Development of intracranial tuberculomas while receiving therapy for pulmonary tuberculosis. Am J Respir Crit Care Med 1994;150:1439–1340.

PATIENT 44

A 45-year-old woman who developed hearing loss during treatment
for tuberculosis

A 45-year-old woman was admitted for treatment of multidrug-resistant tuberculosis. She had been intermittently treated for tuberculosis during the previous 3 years with various regimens that had included several months of streptomycin. Poor compliance had resulted in the emergence of a multidrug-resistant strain. During the preceding 3 months, she had been treated by her primary physician with a regimen consisting of ciprofloxacin, cycloserine, kanamycin, and amoxicillin-clavulanic acid. She denied fever, cough, weight loss, or night sweats, but did complain of severe bilateral hearing loss over the past month. Her most recent drug susceptibility tests revealed tuberculosis resistant to all first-line drugs as well as to ethionamide.

Physical Examination: Vital signs: normal. General: comfortable. Ears: markedly reduced hearing bilaterally. Chest: reduced breath sounds throughout the left lung. Cardiac: normal. Abdomen: no organomegaly.

Laboratory Findings: Hct 34%, WBC 12,000/μl, platelets 114,000/μl. Electrolytes: normal, BUN 13 mg/dl, creatinine 1.0 mg/dl. Chest radiograph: extensive cavitation and infiltrates in the left lung. Audiogram: moderate hearing loss in all frequencies in both ears.

Questions: What is the cause of the hearing loss? What are reasonable treatment recommendations for this patient?

Diagnosis: Aminoglycoside ototoxicity requiring discontinuation of kanamycin.

Discussion: The aminoglycosides streptomycin, kanamycin, and amikacin represent a class of antibiotics that have good activity against *Mycobacterium tuberculosis* but present considerable risks for eighth nerve and renal toxicity. Streptomycin is the preferred first-line aminoglycoside for use in antituberculous regimens because it is less toxic and generally better tolerated than the other aminoglycosides. Nevertheless, eighth nerve injury due to streptomycin occurs in up to 10% of patients and presents most commonly as vestibular dysfunction. Because the risk of ototoxicity is related to cumulative dose, most experts recommend limiting the total dose of streptomycin to less than 120 g.

Decreased hearing may result from therapy with any of the aminoglycosides, but kanamycin is the most common offending agent. Patients initiating aminoglycoside therapy for tuberculosis should be evaluated with baseline audiometry with repeat studies on a monthly basis. Tinnitus may be the first manifestation of eighth nerve damage noticed by the patient. Any manifestations of ototoxicity require discontinuation of aminoglycosides because eighth nerve dysfunction due to these agents is largely irreversible. In patients with multidrug-resistant tuberculosis and severe pulmonary disease, aminoglycosides frequently represent the mainstay of treatment when few other therapeutic options exist. In this setting, clinicians are often faced with the difficult choice of stopping an effective drug long before the treatment course is completed versus subjecting the patient to a continually increasing risk of permanent nerve damage.

Nephrotoxicity can also occur in patients undergoing antituberculous treatment with aminoglycosides. Avoidance of dehydration is an important measure to limit the incidence of this complication of therapy. Patients should be monitored with monthly determinations of serum BUN and creatinine in addition to serial urinalyses. Aminoglycoside doses should be appropriately adjusted if a patient has an impaired creatinine clearance before starting therapy. If abnormalities of renal function develop, the drugs should be decreased or discontinued. Fortunately, the renal side effects are almost always reversible. Less common side effects that may also interfere with therapy include neuromuscular blockade and hypersensitivity reactions.

Although capreomycin is usually grouped with the second-line aminoglycosides, it is actually a polypeptide and is structurally unrelated. This structrural dissimilarity accounts for the absence of cross-resistance between capreomycin and the aminoglycosides. Capreomycin does, however, have the same range of toxicities as the aminoglycosides.

The present patient had suffered severe hearing loss as a result of aminoglycoside use, particularly in the frequency range of normal conversation. After discontinuing the patient's kanamycin, a pneumonectomy was recommended because of the extensive nature of the left-sided infection and the absence of an effective drug regimen for the patient's multidrug-resistant strain. The patient refused surgery, and is currently being treated with ciprofloxacin, cycloserine, para-aminosalicylic acid, clofazimine, and amoxicillin-clavulanic acid. Her sputum smears converted to negative after 2 months of this regimen.

Clinical Pearls

1. The aminoglycosides and capreomycin can produce eighth nerve damage and impaired renal function. Patients undergoing therapy with these agents should be monitored monthly for alterations in auditory, vestibular, and renal function.

2. Because the ototoxicity of aminoglycosides is related to cumulative dose, use of these agents should be limited whenever possible to the first 2–3 months of treatment. The total dose of streptomycin should be less than 120 g.

3. Capreomycin is not technically an aminoglycoside, although it shares their efficacy and toxicities. Cross-resistance between capreomycin and the aminoglycosides does not occur.

REFERENCES

1. Nakayama M, Miura H, Kamei T. Investigation of vestibular damage by antituberculous drugs. Acta Otolaryngol 1991;481:481–485.
2. Donald PR, Doherty E, Van Zyl FJ. Hearing loss in the child following streptomycin administration during pregnancy. Central Afr J Med 1991;37:268–271.
3. Kastanioudakis J, Skevas A, Assimakopoulos D, Anastasopoulos D. Hearing loss and vestibular dysfunction in childhood from the use of streptomycin in Albania. Int J Ped Otorhinolaryngol 1993;26:109–115.
4. Moore RD, Smith CR, Lipsky JJ, et al. Risk factors for nephrotoxicity in patients with aminoglycosides. Ann Intern Med 1984; 100:352–357.

PATIENT 45

A 62-year-old woman with sputum cultures growing *M. fortuitum*

A 62-year-old woman who had recently immigrated to the United States from the Philippines presented with intermittently productive cough and a 15-pound weight loss over the previous 3 months. She denied fevers, chills, and hemoptysis. One month earlier, another physician prescribed 10 days of oral antibiotics, which the patient felt had helped her symptoms somewhat. The patient had no other medical history, took no medications, and did not smoke.

Physical Examination: Temperature 100.3°F, pulse 104, respirations 20. Chest: bronchial breath sounds left upper lung zone. Remainder of the examination was normal.

Laboratory Findings: Hct 43%, WBC 8,950/μl, Electrolytes, liver function tests: normal. Chest radiograph and CT scan: shown below. Sputum: smear negative for acid-fast bacilli, 3 cultures positive for *M. fortuitum.*

Question: What is the best course of treatment for this patient?

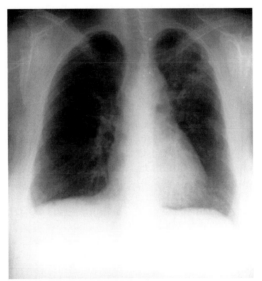

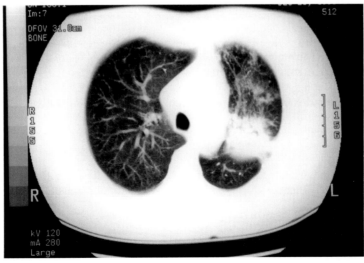

Diagnosis: Lung infection with *Mycobacterium fortuitum.*

Discussion: Mycobacterium fortuitum is a member of the group of organisms known as rapidly growing mycobacteria, so named because they characteristically produce visible colonies on routine culture media in less than 7 days. *M. chelonei* is the other organism in this group that causes disease in humans. Although the organisms can be found in all areas of the country, the majority of cases are concentrated in the southeastern United States. The rapidly growing mycobacteria most commonly cause cutaneous disease, usually following trauma that breaks the skin. Pulmonary disease is far less common, although reports of lung infection with these organisms have been increasing in recent years. Disseminated disease occurs in immunocompromised hosts.

Pulmonary disease due to *M. fortuitum* is typically indolent and insidious in onset. Most patients are white, female, nonsmokers over the age of 50, without underlying lung disease. Almost all patients have cough as the primary symptom. Mild weight loss and low-grade fevers are not uncommon. Exacerbations lasting several weeks may be separated by symptom-free intervals of several months. The chest radiograph usually reveals upper lobe infiltrates, often bilateral, with an interstitial, alveolar, or reticulonodular pattern. Cavitation is uncommon, but bronchiectasis may be seen, particularly if high-resolution CT scans are obtained. As with other nontuberculous mycobacteria, diagnosis is made on the basis of multiple sputum cultures in the absence of other more probable diagnoses.

Several issues distinguish treatment of pulmonary disease caused by *M. fortuitum* from that of other mycobacterial disease. The natural history of this disease is slowly progressive over years. In fact radiographic abnormalities may remain stable for months to years, or occasionally improve without specific therapy.

Deaths from pulmonary disease have rarely been reported. This is probably a reflection of the otherwise good health most patients experience.

Both *M. fortuitum* and *M. chelonei* are resistant to all standard antituberculous medications. *M. fortuitum* is susceptible in vitro to a range of other antibiotics, including the sulfonamides, fluoroquinolones, cefoxitin, amikacin, and imipenem. Additionally, about half of isolates are susceptible to doxycycline and minocycline. Although reports of results of therapy are scanty, in general the majority of patients seem to respond to treatment regimens employing two or three of these agents. The optimal number of drugs and duration of treatment are unknown. Thus the decision to treat must be individualized for each patient, as watchful waiting may be appropriate in patients who are minimally symptomatic. Unfortunately, *M. chelonei* causes over 80% of lung disease due to rapidly growing mycobacteria, and this organism is sensitive only to the parenteral agents cefoxitin, amikacin, and imipenem. Although patients may experience short-term benefit from administration of these antibiotics, cure from medical therapy has not been demonstrated. These patients may be better left untreated, although surgical resection may be beneficial in the few patients with sufficiently localized disease.

The present patient elected to undergo drug therapy because she was severely annoyed by the cough and troubled by the thought of leaving the infection untreated. She was admitted to the hospital and given intravenous ciprofloxacin and amikacin for 2 weeks and discharged on oral sulfamethoxazole, ciprofloxacin, and doxycycline. After three months of therapy, her cough was improved, but the chest radiograph was unchanged. She then returned to the Philippines, where she planned to continue taking the oral antibiotics.

Clinical Pearls

1. The rapidly growing mycobacteria, *M. fortuitum* and *M. chelonei,* most commonly cause infections of the skin and soft tissues. They have the potential, however, for rarely causing an indolent lung disease. Most such patients are infected with *M. chelonei.*

2. The typical patient with *M. fortuitum* lung disease is a nonsmoking, healthy white woman in the southeastern United States who presents with noncavitary, minimally progressive infiltrates on a chest radiograph.

3. The rapidly growing mycobacteria are resistant to all standard antituberculous medications.

4. *M. fortuitum* is usually susceptible to antibiotics, including the sulfonamides, fluoroquinolones, cefoxitin, amikacin, and imipenem, although no treatment may be necessary in many patients.

5. No effective, practical therapy is currently available for pulmonary disease due to *M. chelonei.*

REFERENCES

1. Wallace RJ. The clinical presentation, diagnosis, and therapy of cutaneous and pulmonary infections due to the rapidly growing mycobacteria, *M. fortuitum* and *M. chelonei*. Clin Chest Med 1989;10:419–429.
2. American Thoracic Society. Diagnosis and treatment of disease caused by nontuberculous mycobacteria. Am Rev Respir Dis 1990;142:940–953.
3. Burns DN, Rohatgi PK, Rosenthal R, et al. Disseminated *Mycobacterium fortuitum* successfully treated with combination therapy including ciprofloxacin. Am Rev Respir Dis 1990;142:468–470.
4. Griffith DE, Girard WM, Wallace RJ. Clinical features of pulmonary disease caused by rapidly growing mycobacteria: an analysis of 154 patients. Am Rev Respir Dis 1993;147:1271–1278.

PATIENT 46

A 38-year-old man with abdominal pain and a past history of pulmonary tuberculosis

A 38-year-old man presented to the hospital complaining of abdominal pain. He had a history of pulmonary tuberculosis 15 years prior to admission for which he received three drugs for "many months," according to the patient. Several years prior to admission he had developed a peptic ulcer that had been treated with antacids and H_2-receptor blockade. He had then been well until 2 weeks prior to admission when he developed nausea and diffuse, vague, abdominal pain, without cramping or diarrhea. He denied cough, sputum production, or weight loss.

Physical Examination: Vital signs: normal. General: comfortable. Head: normal. Chest: normal. Heart: normal, without murmurs or rubs. Abdomen: soft, mild right upper quadrant tenderness, liver span 11 cm by percussion, no fluid wave or shifting dullness. Extremities: normal. Neurologic: normal.

Laboratory Findings: CBC and electrolytes: normal. Alanine aminotransferase (SGPT) 176 IU/L, aspartate aminotransferase (SGOT) 257 IU/L, other liver function tests normal. Hepatitis B serologies: antigen and antibody negative. HIV antibody: negative. Chest radiograph: bilateral apical pleural thickening. Liver biopsy: granulomas without acid-fast organisms.

Question: What is the cause of this patient's abdominal complaints and abnormal liver function tests?

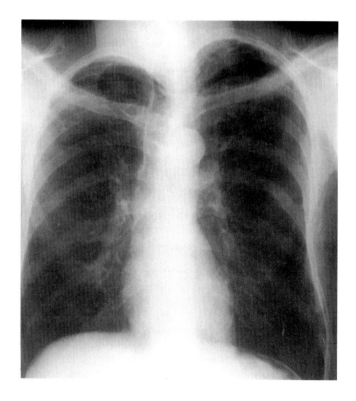

Diagnosis: Granulomatous hepatitis due to infection with *Mycobacterium tuberculosis*.

Discussion: The combination of abdominal pain and abnormal liver function tests in a patient with known or suspected tuberculosis presents a broad differential diagnosis. The most common conditions to be considered, however, include hepatic involvement with tuberculosis, a drug reaction to an antituberculous medication, viral hepatitis, or a toxic hepatitis from alcohol of other exogenous agents. Toxic hepatitis requires careful consideration because of the frequent overlap of alcoholism and tuberculosis in the same patient population, especially those from an urban setting. In the absence of a clear diagnosis for the cause of the abnormal liver function tests, a liver biopsy may be indicated to exclude tuberculous liver disease.

The finding of granulomatous hepatitis on a liver biopsy specimen presents another differential diagnosis that includes direct hepatic involvement by *M. tuberculosis*. The incidence of tuberculosis as a cause of granulomatous hepatitis varies in relation to the prevalence of tuberculosis in the population being evaluated. For example, the percentage of patients with granulomatous hepatitis due to tuberculosis is 3% in the upper midwestern of the United States, a relatively low prevalence region for tuberculosis, and 32% in the Middle East, where tuberculosis is much more common. In Australia, only 6% of patients with granulomatous hepatitis have tuberculosis as the underlying cause. Most instances of this disorder in Australia and the United States, which have similar demographics and levels of economic development, are related to sarcoidosis and idiopathic causes. In Saudia Arabia, however, the most common cause of granulomatous hepatitis is schistosomiasis, which accounts for 54% of patients with the disease.

Asymptomatic liver involvement commonly occurs in patients with pulmonary tuberculosis, but only a minority of patients have abnormalities of their liver function tests. Up to 63% of patients with pulmonary tuberculosis who undergo liver biopsies will have histopathologic abnormalities (granulomas in 18%, nonspecific inflammation in 25%, Kupffer cell hyperplasia in 11%), but only 7% of these patients will demonstrate abnormal liver function tests. The most common abnormalities observed are alterations in SGOT and SGPT. Clinically apparent, isolated granulomatous hepatitis is even less commonly observed as a manifestation of tuberculosis.

The histopathologic findings of granulomatous hepatitis on a liver biopsy specimen require exclusion of tuberculosis from sarcoidosis and idiopathic causes of the disease. Special tissue stains for acid-fast organisms and culturing of the tissue for mycobacteria assist in making this determination, but other tests are also available to the clinician. In a small series of patients with AIDS and hepatic tuberculosis, liver ultrasound abnormalities were noted. These abnormalities included an echogenically "bright" liver, other focal liver lesions, and hypo- or hyperechoic regions. These findings may prove to be nonspecific, but might assist in guiding the biopsy needle to regions of the liver that will have abnormal histopathologic findings. Once diagnosed, hepatic tuberculosis is treated in the same way as pulmonary tuberculosis with antituberculous agents guided by the sensitivity profile of the isolates. In the absence of a liver abscess due to mycobacteria, most patients respond well to therapy.

The present patient was found to have hepatic tuberculosis by the results of the liver biopsy culture, which grew *M. tuberculosis* sensitive to all medications. Presumably, the granulomatous hepatitis represented a relapse of the patient's previous tuberculosis. He was treated with a standard antituberculosis regimen with excellent clinical and laboratory response. The liver biopsy was not repeated.

Clinical Pearls

1. Patients with known or suspected tuberculosis who present with liver function test abnormalities should be evaluated for viral and toxic hepatitis, adverse reactions to drugs, and hepatic tuberculosis.

2. Although histopathologic abnormalities in the liver are frequent findings in patients with pulmonary tuberculosis, clinically apparent hepatic disease does not commonly occur.

3. In developed countries, tuberculosis is an uncommon cause of granulomatous hepatitis. Tuberculosis should be considered, however, in patients who present with granulomatous hepatitis from developing countries where tuberculosis accounts for more than 50% of the patients with the disease.

4. Demonstration of mycobacteria, by direct staining or culture, is required for a diagnosis of tuberculous granulomatous hepatitis.

REFERENCES

1. Anderson CS, Nicholls J, Rowland R, LaBrooy JT. Hepatic granulomas: a 15-year experieince in the Royal Adelaide Hospital. Med J Austral 1988;148:71–74.
2. Sartin JS, Walker RC. Granulomatous hepatitis: a retrospective review of 88 cases at the Mayo Clinic. Mayo Clin Proc 1991;66:914–918.
3. Wetton CW, McCarty M, Tomlinson D, et al. Ultrasound findings in hepatic mycobacterial disease in patients with acquired immunodeficiency syndrome (AIDS). Clin Radiol 1993;47:36–38.
4. Gupta S, Meena HS, Chopra R. Hepatic involvement in tuberculosis. J Assoc Physicians India 1993;41:20–22.

PATIENT 47

An asymptomatic 39-year-old HIV-infected man with a positive tuberculin skin test

A 39-year-old man presented for evaluation of a positive response to a tuberculin skin test that had been placed as a part of his routine health maintenance. He was known to be HIV-infected, but he had no history of opportunistic infection and had recently felt well. His CD4+ cell count had not been measured. There was no history of tuberculosis exposure.

Physical Examination: Vital signs: normal. General: well-nourished, comfortable. The remainder of the examination was normal.

Laboratory Findings: CBC, electrolytes, liver function tests: normal. Tuberculin skin test: 7 mm of induration. Chest radiograph (shown below).

Questions: How should the tuberculin skin test be interpreted? What should be done for this patient?

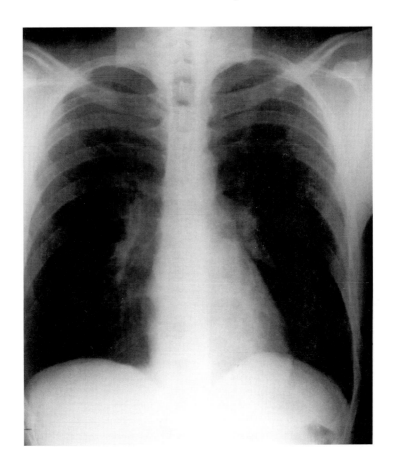

Diagnosis: Tuberculosis infection in an HIV-infected patient.

Discussion: Of all underlying conditions that increase the risk of developing active tuberculosis in a patient with asymptomatic tuberculosis infection, none is more important than HIV infection. In a landmark study, Selwyn and colleagues from Montefiore Medical Center in the Bronx, New York prospectively followed a cohort of tuberculin-positive intravenous drug abusers enrolled in a methadone maintenance program. Similar rates of tuberculin skin test positivity were found in HIV-positive and HIV-negative groups. Skin test responders were followed for 2 years to determine the rate of development of active tuberculosis. Active tuberculosis developed in 8% of the HIV-positive tuberculin responders and none of the HIV-negative responders. Interestingly, only one case of active tuberculosis developed among HIV-positive persons who had a negative tuberculin skin test. The rate of development of active tuberculosis, therefore, was 7.9 per 100 person-years in HIV-positive, tuberculin-positive patients compared to 0.3 per 100 person-years in HIV-positive, tuberculin-negative patients. The major finding of this study, that tuberculin-positive patients infected with HIV are at extraordinarily high risk of developing active tuberculosis, has been corroborated many times. Epidemiologic data from New York City indicate that between 40 and 60% of all cases of active tuberculosis occur in patients seropositive for HIV.

There is now widespread agreement that an HIV-infected patient with a positive tuberculin skin test should receive isoniazid preventive therapy for 12 months regardless of age. However, several circumstances unique to patients with HIV require comment. It is the recommendation of the American Thoracic Society and the Centers for Disease Control and Prevention that 5 mm or more of induration constitutes a positive tuberculin test for patients with HIV infection and indicates the need for isoniazid preventive therapy. This recommendation derives from the impaired delayed-type hypersensitivity response manifested by AIDS patients, who may be able to mount only a weak skin test response to tuberculin testing when they have very low CD4+ cell counts and advanced HIV disease. This situation underlines the importance of performing tuberculin skin testing as early as possible in the course of a patient's HIV infection because preservation of delayed-type hypersensitivity reactions is directly related to the CD4+ T-cell count.

The recommendation for isoniazid prophylaxis in patients with HIV infection and positive tuberculin tests is based on limited data. A problem with this recommendation is the long duration of therapy in a patient population at high risk for progressive disease and poor drug compliance. A controlled trial of preventive therapy comparing 12 months of isoniazid with 2 months of rifampin and pyrazinamide is nearing completion, and results from this study should be available in the near future.

Before an HIV-infected patient is placed on isoniazid preventive therapy, active tuberculosis must be excluded. This is a challenging task because patients with AIDS may have only minimally abnormal or even normal chest radiographs in the presence of active disease. Even minor respiratory symptoms should prompt an aggressive evaluation for pulmonary tuberculosis. If isoniazid alone is given to a patient with active disease, it is likely that a resistant strain will emerge, making the tuberculosis more difficult to treat.

Finally, the use of rifabutin as prophylaxis against disease caused by the *Mycobacterium avium–intracellulare* (MAI) complex of organisms raises issues for which there are no clear answers. Rifabutin (ansamycin) is a relative of rifampin that has been shown to be effective in reducing morbidity from MAI in AIDS patients with CD4+ cell counts less than $100/\mu l$. Because isolates of *M. tuberculosis* that are sensitive to rifampin are usually sensitive to rifabutin, it is logical to consider that tuberculin-positive patients with HIV infection who are being treated with rifabutin may not require additional isoniazid prophylaxis. Few if any data are available, however, regarding the use of either rifampin or rifabutin for tuberculosis prophylaxis. The decision to add isoniazid preventive therapy in a patient on rifabutin, therefore, requires individualization and careful patient follow-up. Furthermore, concerns exist regarding the possibility of generating strains of *M. tuberculosis* resistant to rifampin by the broad use of rifabutin for MAI prophylaxis. This concern underscores the need to exclude active pulmonary tuberculosis in patients about to receive preventive therapy for infections as well as for *M. tuberculosis.*

The present patient had a positive tuberculin test with greater than 5 mm of induration and a normal chest radiograph. Sputum cultures were negative for *M. tuberculosis.* He was treated with 12 months of isoniazid prophylaxis.

Clinical Pearls

1. Patients with HIV infection constitute an extremely high-risk group for development of tuberculosis. Tuberculin testing should be routinely performed in this patient population early in the course of HIV disease.

2. Induration of 5 mm or greater should be interpreted as a positive tuberculin response in patients with HIV infection.

3. Care should be taken to exclude active tuberculosis in any HIV-positive patient who is to be placed on preventive therapy for either *M. tuberculosis* or MAI complex disease.

REFERENCES

1. Chaparas SD, Vandiviere HM, Melvin I, et al. Tuberculin test: variability with the Mantoux procedure. Am Rev Respir Dis 1985;132:175–177.
2. Selwyn PA, Hartel D, Lewis VA, et al. A prospective study of the risk of tuberculosis among intravenous drug users with human immunodeficiency virus infection. N Engl J Med 1989;320:545–550.
3. Bayer R, Dubler NN, Landesman S. The dual epidemics of tuberculosis and AIDS: ethical and policy issues in screening and treatment. Am J Public Health 1993;83:649–654.
4. Markowitz N, Hansen NI, Wilkosky TC, et al. Tuberculin and anergy testing in HIV-seropositive and HIV-seronegative persons: pulmonary complications of HIV infection study group. Ann Intern Med 1993;119:185–193.
5. American Thoracic Society. Treatment of tuberculosis and tuberculosis infection in adults and children. Am J Respir Crit Care Med 1994;149:1359–1375.

PATIENT 48

A 71-year-old HIV-negative woman with pulmonary tuberculosis and CD4+ cell lymphopenia

A 71-year-old woman presented complaining of fever, cough, and weight loss. She was born in China but had immigrated to the United States over 40 years earlier. The patient denied risk factors for HIV infection, specifically denying any surgical procedures or blood transfusions.

Physical Examination: Temperature 101.4°F, pulse 88, respirations 18, blood pressure 110/70. General: ill-appearing, thin, elderly woman. HEENT: normal. Chest: diffuse crackles in all lung fields. Cardiac: normal. Abdomen: normal.

Laboratory Findings: CBC, electrolytes, liver function tests: normal. Chest radiograph: extensive infiltrates throughout all lung fields. Sputum smears: numerous acid-fast bacilli. CD4+ (T-helper) cell count: 165/μl. CD8+ (T-suppresser) cell count: 213/μl. CD4/CD8 ratio = 0.77. Testing for antibodies to HIV was negative on three occasions over 8 weeks.

Question: What is the explanation of the low CD4+ cell count and the reversal of the CD4/CD8 ratio?

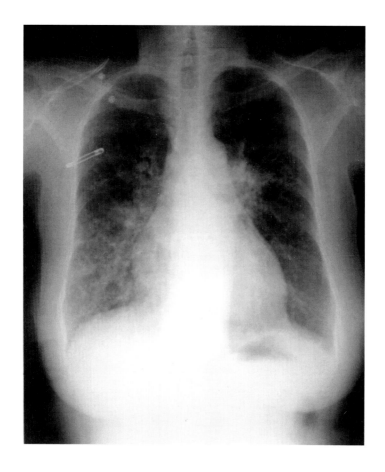

Diagnosis: CD4+ (T-helper) lymphopenia in a patient with active tuberculosis.

Discussion: The host response against intracellular pathogens, such as *M. tuberculosis,* involves a complex and fascinating array of interactions between immune effector cells, cytokine networks, and the offending pathogen. It has long been believed that the key immune cell in the killing of intracellular pathogens in the lung, such as mycobacteria, is the alveolar macrophage, which first engulfs and then kills organisms that reach the peripheral airways. Numerous cytokines, most notably interferon-gamma, play a fundamentally important role in this process by stimulating macrophage generation of reactive nitrogen metabolites that digest intracellular bacteria. Interferon-gamma itself is released largely by lymphocytes of the CD4+ (T-helper) phenotype. These lymphocytic cell lines, therefore, are central initiators of the cytokine-macrophage response that prevents the ability of *M. tuberculosis* to become established in the lung.

Patients with HIV infection are at markedly increased risk of developing tuberculosis partly because of viral-induced suppression of CD4+ lymphocytes with resulting depression of circulating levels of interferon-gamma. Also, HIV can infect alveolar macrophages directly, altering their phagocytic and bacteria-killing capacity. Patients with HIV infection, therefore, have decreased host defenses against intracellular bacterial pathogens such as *M. tuberculosis.*

Interestingly, infection with *M. tuberculosis* even in the absence of HIV disease has been associated with altered host defenses and decreased cellular immunity. Peripheral lymphopenia, for instance, has been noted occasionally in patients with tuberculosis, especially those with advanced, untreated disease. Several investigations suggest that this finding is associated with a poor clinical outcome. In a regression analysis of several clinical and laboratory parameters associated with tuberculosis, one study found that lymphopenia, advanced age, concomitant extrapulmonary tuberculosis, alcoholism, a high peripheral neutrophil count, and lack of cavitation were strongly associated with a poor outcome. It remains unclear, however, whether lymphopenia is a secondary manifestation of tuberculosis or represents an underlying disorder that promotes the onset and progression of the disease.

More recently, investigators reported the occurrence of CD4+ lymphopenia in tuberculosis patients but could not correlate this finding with poor outcome, even in patients with reversal of the CD4/CD8 ratio. Another report described T-cell subsets in 26 patients with newly diagnosed HIV-negative and tuberculosis compared to 29 healthy controls. This report found that CD4+ cell counts were generally lower in patients with tuberculosis ($748/\mu l$ vs. $1043/\mu l$), but the CD4/CD8 ratios were lower than 1.2 in only 6 patients. CD4+ lymphopenia did not seem to correlate with radiographic extent of disease. These investigators suggested that CD4+ lymphopenia was a reaction to mycobacterial disease rather than a manifestation of underlying immunodeficiency. Other workers have demonstrated that a functional defect in T-lymphocytes may exist in patients with tuberculosis, in that interferon-gamma production in patients with tuberculosis was found to be lower in response to certain stimulants than in controls.

The clinical meaning of peripheral lymphopenia in patients with tuberculosis remains ill defined. Future investigations may offer hope that manipulations of the immune system may be helpful in treating patients with active disease. It is clear that lymphopenia, specifically CD4+ lymphopenia, occurs so commonly in patients with tuberculosis that these findings cannot serve as surrogate markers for HIV infection. HIV status should always be confirmed directly with the appropriate serologic studies.

The present patient was considered to have CD4+ lymphopenia as a manifestation of active tuberculosis. No evidence of HIV infection was present. She was treated with isoniazid, ethambutol, pyrazinamide, and rifampin with subsequent adjustment of therapy when her sputum cultures demonstrated a pan-sensitive strain. Two months after initiating therapy, her CD4+ and CD8+ cell counts increased to $1098/\mu l$ and $838/\mu l$, respectively, with a CD4/CD8 ratio of 1.3. She completed her course of therapy without complications.

Clinical Pearls

1. Lymphopenia is a common finding in patients with tuberculosis and has been associated with a poor outcome in a study using multivariate regression analysis.

2. Specific CD4+ lymphopenia with a reversal of the peripheral CD4/CD8 ratio may also occur in patients with tuberculosis. These findings generally normalize during drug therapy for the tuberculous infection.

3. CD4+ lymphopenia in patients with tuberculosis is not necessarily a sign of underlying immunosuppression, and should not be used as a surrogate marker of HIV infection.

REFERENCES

1. Beck JS, Potts RC, Kardjito T, Grange JW. T4 lymphopenia in patients with active pulmonary tuberculosis. Clin Exp Immunol 1985;60:49–54.
2. Onwubalili JK, Edwards AJ, Palmer L. T4 lymphopenia in human tuberculosis. Tubercle 1987;68:195–200.
3. Laurence J. T-cell subsets in health, infectious disease, and idiopathic CD4+ T lymphopenia. Ann Intern Med 1993;119:55–62.
4. Ashtekar MD, Samuel AM, Kadival GV, et al. T lymphocytes in pulmonary tuberculosis. Indian J Med Res 1993;97:14–17.
5. Turett GS, Telzak EE. Normalization of CD4+ T-lymphocyte depletion in patients without HIV infection treated for tuberculosis. Chest 1994;105:1335–1337.

PATIENT 49

A 38-year-old hospital employee with a positive tuberculin skin test 2 weeks after an initial negative test

A 38-year-old new hospital employee was referred for evaluation of a positive tuberculin skin test. The patient had an initial tuberculin test placed 3 weeks earlier as part of routine pre-employment health screen. The skin test was negative but a repeat tuberculin test 2 weeks later was positive with 10 mm of induration. The patient felt well and denied contact with any persons with known tuberculosis. He denied HIV risk factors and stated that he had never been tuberculin tested before.

Physical Examination: Vital signs: normal. General: appeared healthy. The remainder of the examination was normal.

Laboratory Findings: CBC, serum electrolytes, liver function tests: normal. Chest radiograph: normal.

Questions: How should the patient's tuberculin skin test results be interpreted? What therapy, if any, should be prescribed?

Diagnosis: Positive tuberculin skin test elicited by two-step tuberculin skin testing.

Discussion: Tuberculin skin testing with purified protein derivative (PPD) remains the only practical test that is useful on a large scale basis for detecting tuberculosis infection. Because interpretation of the test is not always straightforward, however, tuberculin skin testing as a screening tool should be limited to well-defined circumstances. Tuberculin screening programs should primarily focus on known contacts of persons with active tuberculosis, individuals at extremely high risk of developing tuberculosis (AIDS, prolonged therapy with immunosuppressive drugs), and individuals such as hospital or nursing home employess, who could transmit the disease to a large number of vulnerable persons. Persons at high risk for recent tuberculosis infection (immigrants from countries with a high prevalence of tuberculosis) and persons with radiographic abnormalities suggestive of old untreated tuberculosis should also undergo tuberculin skin testing.

Interpretation of a skin test result depends on the clinical circumstances of the patient: 5 mm of induration (not erythema) is considered positive for patients with HIV infection, close contacts of active tuberculosis cases, and persons with chest radiographs suggestive of previous tuberculosis; 10 mm of induration is considered positive in injection drug users, persons from tuberculosis endemic areas, medically underserved populations, persons with medical conditions associated with an increased risk of tuberculosis, and residents of long-term care facilities, including prisons; and 15 mm of induration is considered positive for all other persons.

In most instances, tuberculin skin testing need be performed only once for any given individual. Health care workers, however, should undergo annual or semi-annual testing to monitor an institution's infection control practices and to provide maximal protection of employees from occupational tuberculosis. In programs where individuals will be tested repeatedly, two-step testing is recommended if the first tuberculin skin test is negative. This procedure is recommended to detect the presence of the **booster phenomenon.**

The booster effect represents an immunologic response to an initial exposure to PPD. When widespread tuberculin skin testing first came into use, it was recognized that some persons known to be infected with tuberculosis had lost skin test reactivity to PPD over several years. When such persons were rechallenged with PPD within 2–4 weeks after a negative test, however, skin test reactivity became reestablished. Presumably, the second test "boosts" or stimulates the response of certain T-lymphocytes to restore the delayed hypersensitivity response characteristic of latent tuberculosis infection.

In interpreting the booster response, it should be recognized that the first test is a false negative and the second (boosted) test is a true positive. If the booster phenomenon is unrecognized and unaccounted for in interpreting skin tests, many persons will be misclassified as new converters if the second test is performed one or more years later and will be mistakenly prescribed isoniazid preventive therapy. This risk for misinterpretation underlies the recommendation to perform two-step tuberculin testing for individuals with an initial negative skin test if such persons are to be assessed on a regular basis for tuberculosis infection. It is important to note that both of the tuberculin skin tests should be performed with 0.1 ml of 5TU PPD injected intradermally.

The present health care worker's second skin test was interpreted as a boosted, true-positive result, indicative of previous tuberculosis infection. Because his chest radiograph was normal and he was not known to be a new converter, a close contact of an active case, HIV seropositive, or otherwise at increased risk for developing active tuberculosis, isoniazid preventive therapy was not recommended.

Clinical Pearls

1. Tuberculin skin testing should be applied only to targeted groups who have risk factors for tuberculosis infection or who, if they developed active disease, could transmit the disease to many other individuals.

2. Criteria for a positive tuberculin skin test vary with the clinical characteristics of the patient being tested. Importantly, 5 mm of induration is indicative of a positive test in a person with HIV infection.

3. For persons who will undergo tuberculin skin testing on an annual or semi-annual basis, two-step testing should be performed if the initial test is negative, in order to account for the booster phenomenon and to prevent misclassification of previously infected persons as new converters.

REFERENCES

1. Slutkin G, Perez-Stable EJ, Hopewell PC. Time course and boosting of tuberculin reactions in nursing home residents. Am Rev Respir Dis 1986;134:1048–1051.
2. Havlir DV, van der Kuyp F, Duffy E, et al. A 19-year follow-up of tuberculin reactors: assessment of a skin test reactivity and in vitro lymphocyte responses. Chest 1991;99:1172–1176.
3. American Thoracic Society. Control of tuberculosis in the United States. Am Rev Respir Dis 1992;146:1623–1633.
4. Menzies R, Vissandjee B, Rocher I, St. Germain Y. The booster effect in two-step tuberculin testing among young adults in Montreal. Ann Intern Med 1994;120:190–198.

PATIENT 50

A 44-year-old woman with treated tuberculosis and hemoptysis

A 44-year-old woman with a history of fully treated pulmonary tuberculosis 14 years earlier presented with a cough of 2 weeks' duration. The cough had originally been nonproductive, but over the past 2 days she had coughed up approximately one cup of bloody sputum containing some hard, white particles. She denied fever, chills, weight loss, or chest pain.

Physical Examination: Normal.

Laboratory Findings: CBC and electrolytes: normal. Chest radiograph: below top. CT: below bottom.

Question: What is the likely cause of this woman's hemoptysis?

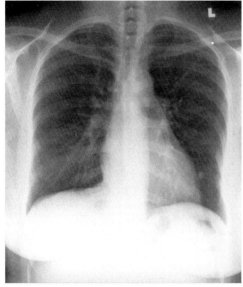

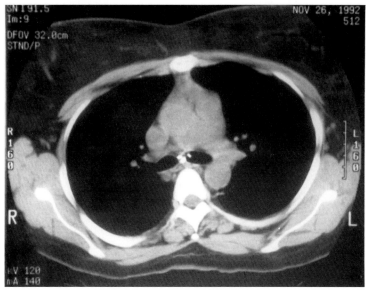

Diagnosis: Broncholithiasis secondary to a previous tuberculous infection.

Discussion: The term broncholithiasis describes a clinical condition in which calcified peribronchial lymph nodes protrude into the airways (broncholiths), occasionally causing patients to expectorate (lithoptysis) "rock-like" nodal fragments. The adenopathy most commonly results from an infectious, granulomatous process that causes dystrophic calcification. Although tuberculosis and histoplasmosis are the most common causes of broncholithiasis, nodal infections associated with coccidioidomycosis and cryptococcosis can also produce this condition. Once calcified, a peribronchial lymph node can erode into a bronchus aided by respiratory motion, which causes the "fixed stone" to abrade the bronchial wall. Rarely, a broncholith may begin as a pulmolith within a region of chronic pulmonary parenchymal infection before working its way proximally into the tracheobronchial tree. Regardless of the etiology, the composition of broncholiths is quite similar to bone, containing 85% calcium phosphate and 15% calcium carbonate.

The signs and symptoms associated with broncolithiasis result from the local mechanical effects on the airway. Virtually all patients have a cough from bronchial irritation. About one-half of patients have hemoptysis, which may be massive if the broncolith erodes through a major vessel adjacent to the airway. Approximately one-quarter of patients will experience lithoptysis, the expectoration of calcified material, which is pathognomonic for this condition. The physical examination is nonspecific, but a localized wheeze or even signs of atelectasis may be noted if sufficient bronchial obstruction is present.

Chest radiographs generally demonstrate little more than calcified lymph nodes, unless airway obstruction with atelectasis has occurred. Infiltrates may reflect partial bronchial obstruction or aspirated blood. The relationship of the calcified particles to the airways is usually not clear unless movement or disappearance of the particles is demonstrated on serial films. CT scans of the chest may be useful in more precisely delineating the association between a calcified node and an airway. The CT can mistakenly show that calcified material is endobronchial when it is not, and, conversely, a true broncholith may appear to be peribronchial rather than endobronchial. These problems are generally due to volume averaging inherent to relatively thick (10 mm) cuts, and can be overcome by the utilization of thin sections (e.g., $\leq$ 2 mm). CT can also demonstrate more subtle associated findings such as bronchiectasis or air trapping (from a partial ball-valve-like obstruction).

The CT scan may also be of use in distinguishing calcified lymphadenopathy from a calcified mediastinal mass, which may represent the more ominous diagnosis of fibrosing medistinitis due to histoplasmosis. Fiberoptic bronchoscopy is generally considered to be complementary to CT in establishing a diagnosis, although only one-half of broncholiths can be visualized endobronchially, limiting the usefulness of bronchoscopy in this disorder.

Complications of broncholithiasis include massive hemoptysis, postobstructive pneumonia, and esophageal perforation. A unique case of a calcified lymph node eroding through the site of anastomosis in a lung transplant patient leading to bronchial dehiscence has been reported. As the majority of patients have no serious complications of broncholithiasis, intervention in the form of broncholithectomy is reserved for patients with recurrent or massive hemoptysis. This can usually be accomplished simply and safely using a rigid bronchoscope, although recurrence from incomplete removal is not uncommon. Thoracotomy is a much more invasive procedure that is usually definitive. Fiberoptic bronchoscopy can usually accomplish little except partial fragmentation of the broncholith with forceps. However, use of a YAG laser via a fiberoptic scope to achieve fragmentation has been reported to facilitate broncholithectomy, and may obviate the need for thoracotomy.

In the present patient, hemoptysis resolved shortly after the lithoptysis occurred. Twelve months later the patient remains asymptomatic except for a mild chronic cough.

Clinical Pearls

1. Lymph nodes involved with prior granulomatous infections such as tuberculosis, histoplasmosis, coccidioidomycosis, or cryptococcosis may calcify and subsequently extrude particles called broncholiths into the airway.

2. CT scan and bronchoscopy are usually complementary in establishing the diagnosis of broncholithiasis, although either or both may not demonstrate the endobronchial location of the broncholith.

3. Common complications of broncholithiasis include hemoptysis (sometimes massive), postobstructive pneumonia, and esophageal perforation.

4. Broncholithectomy by rigid bronchoscopy is indicated in patients with complications, although flexible bronchoscopy and laser therapy are alternative or adjunctive procedures.

REFERENCES

1. Dixon GF, Donnerberg RL, Schonfeld SA, Whitcomb ME. Clinical commentary: advances in the diagnosis and treatment of broncholithiasis. Am Rev Respir Dis 1984;129:1028–1030.
2. Conces DJ Jr., Tarver RD, Vix VA. Broncholithiasis: CT features in 15 patients. AJR 1991;157:249–53.
3. Doud JR, Bakhos M, McCabe MA, Garrity ER Jr. Bronchial dehiscence associated with a large broncholith in a lung transplant recipient. Chest 1992;102:1273–1274.
4. Sexauer WP, Criner GJ. Recurrent hemopytsis, chest pain, and purulent sputum in a young man. Chest 1992;101:1427–1428.

PATIENT 51

A 53-year-old man with AIDS, an upper-lobe cavitary infiltrate, and mediastinal adenopathy

A 53-year-old man with AIDS presented with complaints of fevers, cough, and shortness of breath of 2 weeks' duration. He had been treated for *Pneumocystis carinii* pneumonia (PCP) 3 months earlier, with a full recovery. Since that time he had been taking prophylactic trimethoprim-sulfamethoxazole. His clinic physician ordered a gallium scan, which revealed moderate diffuse uptake throughout both lungs. The patient was then admitted for further evaluation. He denied sputum production, weight loss, or night sweats. He did not know of any exposure to tuberculosis, and thought that his tuberculin status had always been negative. He had moved from Puerto Rico 20 years earlier, and had used intravenous drugs until 6 years previously.

Physical Examination: Temperature 103°F. General: cachectic, awake and alert. Skin: needle track marks. The remainder of the examination was normal.

Laboratory Findings: Hct 36%, WBC 1800/μl. Electrolytes, blood chemistries: normal. Sputum smears: negative for acid-fast bacilli. Skin tests: anergic. CD4+ count: 290/μl. Chest radiograph and CT scan: shown below.

Clinical Course: The patient underwent fiberoptic bronchoscopy to diagnose the cause of the infiltrates. Small pustular lesions about 2–3 mm in diameter were seen diffusely throughout the airways. Endobronchial biopsies of these lesions and transbronchial biopsies in the right upper-lobe infiltrate were performed.

Question: Should this patient have undergone bronchoscopy or received empirical therapy for tuberculosis with careful monitoring for a clinical response?

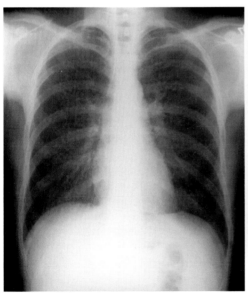
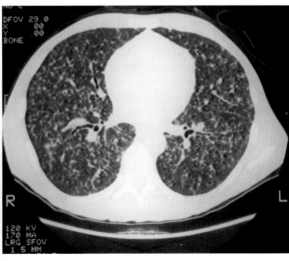

Diagnosis: Disseminated histoplasmosis.

Discussion: Histoplasmosis is a fungus endemic to the Mississippi and Ohio River Valleys as well as Central and South America. Disease in humans occurs when the micronidia or hyphae are inhaled and reach the alveoli, where they germinate into yeast. Because histoplasmosis is a soil-dwelling organism that thrives in a high-nitrogen environment, exposure may be particularly common in areas such as farms, construction and excavation sites, and areas where bird or bat excrement is plentiful, such as chicken coops and caves.

After infection has occurred, alveolar macrophages ingest the organism, and are helped to contain the infection by cell-mediated immunity (CMI). Specifically, T-lymphocytes arm the macrophages, enabling them to kill intracellular organisms. During the early phase of this period, which takes place within 2 weeks of infection, the organism is disseminated by the hematogenous route throughout the body. Nonetheless, infections are either asymptomatic or cause a mild, self-limited, flu-like illness in 99% of patients. Most individuals who become ill either have an acute, self-limited pneumonia after massive exposure, or have defects in CMI, usually from immunosuppressive drugs or from AIDS. Approximately 2–5% of AIDS patients in the United States live in endemic areas, and those who develop histoplasmosis may reactivate a previous infection or develop disease following a new infection. Evidence for both etiologies exists. Some patients have calcified lymph nodes representing remote infection, or have lived in a nonendemic region for years prior to developing disease, whereas others develop disease during an outbreak in a particular area, implying new infection.

Those with CMI defects such as AIDS present with 1–2 months of fever, fatigue, and weight loss. Most have a miliary pattern on chest radiograph, reflecting disseminated disease, although up to 10% may have normal radiographs in this setting. Approximately 20% have evidence of intrathoracic adenopathy. Meningitis, gastrointestinal disease, and skin involvement each occur in about 10–20% of patients. Approximately 10–20% will present severely ill with a sepsis-like syndrome, which has a poor prognosis.

Another presentation that has been described in immunocompetent hosts is that of chronic cavitary histoplasmosis. This is a relatively indolent illness that may present with signs and symptoms similar to those of tuberculosis, usually in older patients with underlying chronic obstructive lung disease. The radiographic findings typically are upper lobe cavities that can slowly progress or may resolve spontaneously.

Diagnosis of histoplasmosis can be challenging. Skin testing is of limited value, as the majority of residents in an endemic area will have positive results, representing a remote, inactive infection. Definitive diagnosis is usually made by culture, which is positive in up to 90% of blood or bone marrow specimens, and up to 75% of bronchoscopic specimens. As cultures may take up to 4 weeks for a positive result, more rapid detection is preferable. The lysis-centrifugation technique for blood cultures may significantly decrease the time course for a positive culture. Even more promising, although not yet widely available, is detection of antigen, which is positive in up to 95% of urine or blood specimens and may provide results within 1 day. Currently, rapid diagnosis is probably made most commonly by detecting the organism through staining of appropriate tissue specimens. While this has an overall sensitivity of about 40%, the yield is highest in bone marrow specimens, up to 75%.

While disseminated histoplasmosis is universally fatal if left untreated in patients with AIDS, a rapid and sustained response to appropriate antifungal therapy is common. About 80% of patients will experience a clinical response within the first week of treatment with amphotericin B, which is the best treatment for all but the most mild cases. As virtually all patients with AIDS will relapse when therapy is discontinued, maintenance therapy, usually with itraconazole, is required for the rest of the patient's life. Metabolism of itraconazole is markedly increased in patients who are also taking rifampin, necessitating an increase in dose.

The present patient achieved a good clinical response to amphotericin B, which he received after all bronchoscopic biopsy specimens revealed numerous organisms morphologically consistent with histoplasmosis. Following administration of a total dose of 1 gm of amphotericin B, he is currently being maintained on itraconazole as suppressive therapy.

Clinical Pearls

1. Histoplasmosis is a soil-dwelling organism to which humans are exposed in areas such as farms, construction and excavation sites, and caves, particularly in the Mississippi and Ohio River Valleys.

2. While 99% of people infected with histoplasmosis are not ill, those with defects in cell-mediated immunity, such as AIDS, are at high risk for developing serious or disseminated disease.

3. Diagnosis is most commonly made by the demonstration of the organism in tissue specimens; antigen detection in urine or blood samples is a rapid and sensitive means of making the diagnosis.

4. Treatment of histoplasmosis in patients with AIDS is usually effective and requires an induction phase using amphotericin B followed by lifelong maintenance with itraconazole.

REFERENCES

1. Salzman SH, Smith RL, Aranda CP. Histoplasmosis in patients at risk for the acquired immunodeficiency syndrome in a nonendemic setting. Chest 1988;93:916–921.
2. Rubin SA, Winer-Muram HT. Thoracic histoplasmosis. J Thorac Imag 1992;7:39–50.
3. Wheat J. Histoplasmosis and coccidiomycosis in individuals with AIDS. Infect Dis Clin North Am 1994;8:467–482.

PATIENT 52

A 46-year-old man with pulmonary tuberculosis and hyponatremia

A 46-year-old man presented to the hospital with a 4-month history of chest pain, cough, and fever. The patient had abused intravenous drugs and alcohol in the past, and had smoked 2 packs of cigarettes a day for 20 years.

Physical Examination: Temperature 101°F, pulse 92, respirations 16, blood pressure 136/84. General: thin, ill-appearing man. Head: normal. Chest: scattered bilateral crackles. Heart: normal heart sounds, without murmurs. Abdomen: normal. Neurologic: normal.

Laboratory Findings: Hct 31%, WBC 10,100/μl. Na$^+$ 121 mEq/L, K$^+$ 3.5 mEq/L, Cl$^-$ 92 mEq/L, HCO$_3^-$ 22 mEq/L. Urine osmolality: 377 mOsm/L. ACTH stimulation test: normal. Chest radiograph: bilateral fibrocavitary infiltrates. Sputum smear: numerous acid-fast bacilli.

Questions: What is the cause of the hyponatremia? How should it be treated?

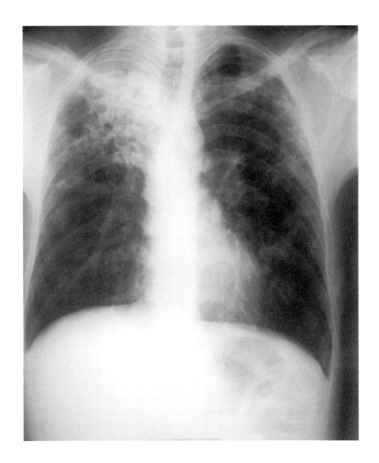

Diagnosis: Syndrome of inappropriate antidiuretic hormone secretion (SIADH) due to pulmonary tuberculosis.

Discussion: The finding of a low serum sodium in a patient who is clinically euvolemic suggests the diagnosis SIADH. It has been well known for many years that SIADH accompanies a variety of lung diseases, including chronic obstructive pulmonary disease, pneumonia, lung abscess, and pulmonary neoplasms, particularly small-cell carcinoma. The syndrome is also common in conjunction with central nervous system disorders such as subdural hematoma and purulent meningitis. Many drugs have been associated with SIADH, including chlorpropamide, vincristine, vinblastine, cyclophosphamide, and tricyclic antidepressants. Both pulmonary tuberculosis and tuberculous meningitis have been associated with SIADH, although the syndrome occurs more commonly in the latter disorder.

The pathophysiology of SIADH is related to an excessive release or enhanced effect on renal tubules of arginine vasopressin. The resultant increased biologic effect of ADH results in hyponatremia, the excretion of inappropriately concentrated urine, and clinically modest degrees of hypervolemia. The exact mechanism for SIADH in patients with tuberculosis is unclear. One investigative group studied 28 hyponatremic patients with pulmonary or miliary tuberculosis. They found that all study subjects exhibited a decline in urine osmolality and an increase in total body free water after a period of water loading. Water excretion was normal, however, in only 7 of 22 subjects, and the remainder showed some impairment of urinary diluting ability. Despite the presence of serum hypo-osmolality that typically lowers circulating vasopressin to below detectable levels, ADH was detectable in 94% of the study subjects; levels declined in a normal direction, however, after water loading. In all of the studied patients, hyponatremia resolved promptly after the institution of antituberculous therapy.

In some conditions, such as small-cell lung cancer, SIADH develops as a consequence of excessive release of vasopressin from an ectopic focus. In tuberculosis, granulomas have been found to be hormonally active. Tuberculous granulomas are known to synthesize 1-α-hydroxylase, which is the enzyme that catalyzes the formation of 1,25-OH vitamin D and thereby leads to hypercalcemia. Some evidence exists that these granulomas can also produce arginine vasopressin, which may cause SIADH.

Patients with tuberculous meningitis may also experience SIADH. In this condition, hyponatremia is more likely to occur in patients with raised rather than normal intracranial pressures. This observation suggests that an increased circulating ADH concentration may be the body's attempt to expand the intravascular space, raise mean arterial pressure, and maintain cerebral perfusion in the face of raised intracranial pressure. In this circumstance, hyponatremia is a secondary event.

The diagnosis of SIADH is suggested by the presence of hyponatremia in a patient who appears clinically euvolemic. Thyroid and adrenal insufficiency must also be excluded because both conditions can cause euvolemic hyponatremia. A measured urine osmolality that is not maximally dilute in the setting of hyponatremia strongly supports the diagnosis. The normal renal response in euvolemic patients with hyponatremia of other causes would be to maximize urinary excretion of free water to resolve the serum dilution of sodium.

The treatment of SIADH depends on the degree of hyponatremia and the seriousness of the patient's clinical manifestations. Alterations of mental status typically dictate aggressive efforts to reverse the hypo-osmolality. Fluid restriction, diuretic therapy, administration of hypertonic saline, and the use of demeclocycline (which creates a type of nephrogenic diabetes insipidus) represent the available interventions that may be appropriate under certain circumstances. In SIADH due to tuberculosis, however, the ultimate treatment is antituberculous therapy.

The absence of symptoms related to plasma hypo-osmolality and the moderate degree of hyponatremia noted in the present patient allowed his physicians to avoid specific interventions to raise the serum sodium. The hyponatremia resolved after the institution of antituberculous therapy.

Clinical Pearls

1. Pulmonary and central nervous system tuberculous are both associated with the syndrome of inappropriate secretion of antidiuretic hormone.

2. In patients with tuberculosis and hyponatremia, adrenal insufficiency should be excluded, since tuberculosis may cause hypoadrenalism, which is also associated with hyponatremia.

3. Response of the hyponatremia to antituberculous therapy in patients with SIADH is the rule.

REFERENCES

1. Hill AR, Uribarri J, Mann J, Berl T. Altered water metabolism in tuberculosis: role of vasopressin. Am J Med 1990;88:357–364.
2. Motiwala HG, Sanghvi NP, Bartjatiya MK, Patel SM. Syndrome of inappropriate antidiuretic hormone following tuberculous epididymo-orchitis in a renal transplant recipient: case report. J Urol 1991;146:1366–1367.
3. Cotton MF, Donald PR, Schoeman JF, et al. Raised intracranial pressure, the syndrome of inappropriate antidiuretic hormone secretion, and arginine vasopressin in tuberculous meningitis. Childs Nerv Syst 1993;9:10–16.

PATIENT 53

A 25-year-old man with partially treated tuberculosis

A 25-year-old man with a history of HIV infection and pulmonary tuberculosis was evaluated for a productive cough and fever of 2 weeks' duration. Four years earlier, the patient initiated therapy with isoniazid, rifampin, and pyrazinamide for a diagnosis of pulmonary tuberculosis. He discontinued therapy after 2 months, and subsequently haphazardly took antituberculous drugs for many short episodes when he presented to physicians with recurrent respiratory symptoms. The patient could could not remember all of the medications he had received, but recalled that multiple different regimens were prescribed, which sometimes included injectable agents.

Physical Examination: Temperature 103.2°F. General: ill-appearing man. Neck: diffuse shotty lymphadenopathy. Chest: bronchial breath sounds in the right upper lobe. Cardiac: normal. Abdomen: normal. Extremities: normal.

Laboratory Findings: Sputum: numerous acid-fast organisms. Chest radiograph (below): cavitary infiltrate in the right upper lobe.

Question: What should be the initial approach to this patient's antituberculous therapy?

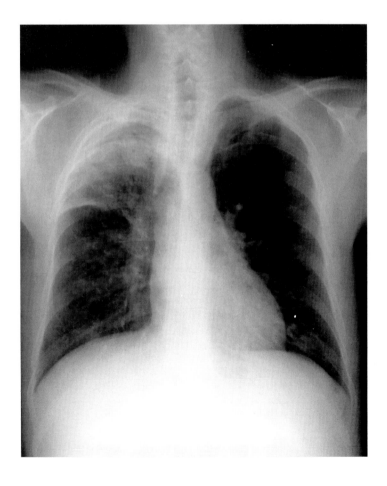

Diagnosis: Active tuberculosis in a patient at high risk for multidrug resistance because of previous erratic administration of drugs.

Discussion: The selection of an adequate combination of antituberculous drugs and an assurance that a patient will comply with a therapeutic regimen remain two of the most important challenges in the successful management of tuberculosis. When a patient presents for the first time with active tuberculosis, choosing an adequate regimen is a relatively simple task. Unless the patient is a close contact of a known case of drug-resistant tuberculosis, initial therapy should include isoniazid, rifampin, and pyrazinamide. Current recommendations stipulate that a fourth drug, either ethambutol or streptomycin, be included in the initial treatment of patients from communities where drug resistance is found in at least 4% of isolates. In communities where resistance to both isoniazid and rifampin is common, it may be preferable to initiate therapy with five or six drugs. Drug susceptibility testing should be performed on all initial positive cultures, with subsequent tailoring of the regimen based on the results.

These therapeutic recommendations derive from the observation that two or more drugs to which the organism is sensitive are required to prevent the emergence of drug resistance. It is often difficult to design a regimen that adheres to this principle in patients who present with active tuberculosis after a period of ineffective drug therapy. In this setting, it is fundamentally important to obtain a full treatment history that includes the drug regimens used, drug susceptibility patterns at the time of treatment, duration of treatment, and response to therapy. Without full knowledge of previous treatment, the physician may unwittingly administer several drugs, of which only one is effective against a resistant organism. This error makes an already resistant organism newly resistant to additional drugs.

Any medications that were part of an inadequate or failing regimen must be considered potentially ineffective when designing a new regimen. When resistance to isoniazid and rifampin is known or suspected, the new regimen should include a minimum of three drugs that the patient has not previously received or to which the organism is known to be sensitive.

The present patient was assumed to be infected with a multidrug-resistant strain of *M. tuberculosis* because of his history of poor compliance with therapy. No medications were administered until a complete drug history was obtained from his previous physicians. Several days later, it was learned that he had received erratic regimens containing isoniazid, rifampin, pyrazinamide, ethambutol, and streptomycin. Sensitivity testing had been performed on only one isolate that had been obtained at the onset of the third course of treatment. That isolate was resistant to isoniazid and rifampin. With this information, treatment was initiated with ciprofloxacin, cycloserine, ethionamide, and kanamycin pending further sensitivity testing. The organism was subsequently found to be resistant to isoniazid, rifampin, ethambutol, and streptomycin (susceptibility testing for pyrazinamide was not available).

Clinical Pearls

1. Drug susceptibility testing should be performed on all initial isolates of *M. tuberculosis,* and repeated when clinical suspicion of new drug resistance arises.

2. A single drug should never be added to a failing antituberculous regimen.

3. Initial drug regimens for tuberculosis should be based on knowledge of the prevailing drug-susceptiblity patterns in the community.

4. When confronted with a patient who has been noncompliant with multiple treatment courses, it is prudent to withhold therapy until the full treatment history and previous drug-susceptiblity patterns are known, unless the patient is at risk of imminent death from tuberculosis.

5. When resistance to isoniazid and rifampin is known or suspected, treatment should include a minimum of three drugs that the patient has not previously received or to which the organism is known to be sensitive.

REFERENCES

1. Mahmoudi A, Iseman MD. Pitfalls in the care of patients with tuberculosis. JAMA 1993;270:65–68.
2. Iseman MD. Treatment of multidrug-resistant tuberculosis. N Engl J Med 1993;329:784–791.
3. Harkin TJ, Harris HW. Treatment of multidrug-resistant tuberculosis. In: Rom WN, Garay SM, eds. Tuberculosis. Boston: Little, Brown, 1995.

PATIENT 54

A 77-year-old woman with dyspnea, fevers, and positive acid-fast sputum smears

A 77-year-old woman with a 3-year history of a productive cough and intermittent fevers presented to the hospital with increasing dyspnea, fevers, and sputum production. She had noted a 15-pound weight loss over the past year. A CT scan of the chest 1 year earlier revealed bronchiectasis. Multiple bouts of increased sputum resolved when the patient was treated with azithromycin. There was no history of exposure to tuberculosis, and a tuberculin skin test had been reported as negative.

Physical Examination: Temperature 101°F. General: frail-appearing elderly woman in no distress. Chest: coarse rhonchi bilaterally. Cardiac: normal. Abdomen: normal. Extremeties: no cyanosis or clubbing.

Laboratory Findings: Hct 34%, WBC 12,000 /μl. Electrolytes: normal. ABG (room air): pH 7.48, PCO_2 41 mmHg, PO_2 65 mmHg. Sputum smear: positive for acid-fast bacilli. Chest radiograph and CT: shown below.

Question: What mycobacterial pathogen is typically present in this clinical setting?

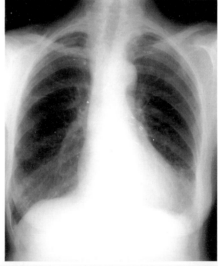

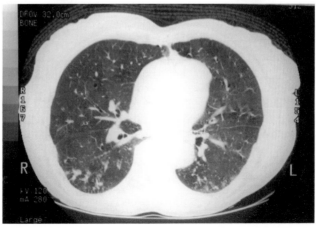

Diagnosis: Mycobacterium avium complex infection with bronchiectasis.

Discussion: Organisms of the *Mycobacterium avium* complex (MAC) occur ubiquitously in soil and water. Although these organisms may colonize the airways of patients with underlying lung disease, they are also well-recognized causes of pulmonary disease in some clinical settings. Two distinct forms of lung disease occur in immunocompetent patients infected with MAC. The first form occurs most often in elderly male smokers who have underlying chronic obstructive lung disease. These patients present with progressive upper-lobe cavities that appear radiographically similar to pulmonary tuberculosis. These patients, however, respond poorly to antituberculous drug regimens. The second form of lung disease develops almost entirely in nonsmoking women who have no radiographic evidence of lung cavities. In contrast to the first form of MAC infection, these patients have a lower organism load in their lungs, as manifested by a lower frequency of positive sputum smears and sputum cultures. Typical radiographic findings include nodular and interstitial infiltrates, often in the right middle lobe or lingula. Early reports of this condition noted an association with bronchiectasis and a nonprogressive course in most patients who were followed with standard radiographs. This stability of the radiographic infiltrates suggested that the MAC organisms were simple colonizers of airways that were preexistingly bronchiectatic.

More recently, however, high-resolution CT (HRCT) scans have more accurately characterized the clinical importance of MAC organisms as pathogens in the second form of MAC infection. These studies demonstrate an association between positive sputum cultures for MAC and the presence of focal bronchiectasis and small pulmonary nodules. These nodules are usually less than 5 mm in diameter and occur adjacent to bronchiectatic airways. HRCT scans have detected progression of these lung abnormalities when patients have been evaluated at intervals of 1–2 years. These observations support the concept that MAC organisms are true pathogens in these patients, and may be the cause rather than the result of the bronchiectasis. Some reports have provided pathologic evidence that the small nodules are granulomas, thereby lending support to the pathogenicity of MAC in these patients.

Although relatively indolent, infection with MAC in women with bronchiectasis may not follow a benign course. One study reported that 4 of 18 patients eventually died as a result of MAC lung disease. Despite the progressive and potentially lethal course of this disease, little data indicate that drug therapy alters the clinical outcome in this condition. Recommendations regarding indications for treatment, drug selection, and duration of therapy are largely empiric. Agents such as clarithromycin, rifabutin, ciprofloxacin, streptomycin, and ethambutol are effective against MAC in vitro, and are probably of benefit in vivo as well. If drug therapy is initiated on the basis of the severity of symptoms and radiographic evidence of progressive disease, at least three or four drugs selected on the basis of drug-susceptibility results should be employed with the expectation of continuing treatment for 18–24 months. All patients with the first form of MAC infection characterized by progressive lung cavities should be treated with the drug regimens described above.

Because of the positive acid-fast sputum smear, the present patient was begun on a standard four-drug antituberculous regimen for a presumptive diagnosis of tuberculosis. These medications were discontinued when the sputum cultures grew MAC organisms. The patient elected not to pursue drug therapy after a discussion of the treatment options with her physician. After a course of vigorous chest physical therapy, the patient's symptoms improved somewhat. Plans were made to follow her with an HRCT scan to be repeated in 1 year.

Clinical Pearls

1. Two distinct syndromes of MAC lung disease exist in immunocompetent hosts: upper lobe cavitary disease in elderly men with COPD, and right middle lobe and lingular nodular infiltrates with bronchiectasis in older women.

2. HRCT may demonstrate the association of bronchiectasis and small parenchymal nodules in women with MAC lung disease. Scans 1–2 years apart may demonstrate disease progression.

3. Patients with the cavitary form of the disease should be treated for 18–24 months with at least three of the following drugs: clarithromycin, rifabutin, ciprofloxacin, streptomycin, or ethambutol.

4. The decision to treat noncavitary disease should be individualized because 3–4 drugs may be required for 24 months or longer, and clinical benefit remains unproven.

REFERENCES

1. Prince DS, Peterson DD, Steiner RM, et al. Infection with *Mycobacterium avium* complex in patients without predisposing conditions. N Engl J Med 1989;321:863–868.
2. American Thoracic Society. Diagnosis and treatment of disease caused by nontuberculous mycobacteria. Am Rev Respir Dis 1990;142:940–953.
3. Reich JM, Johnson RE. *Mycobacterium avium* complex pulmonary disease. Am Rev Respir Dis 1991;143:1381–1385.
4. Swensen SJ, Hartman TE, Williams DE. Computed tomographic diagnosis of *Mycobacterium avium–intracellulare* complex in patients with bronchiectasis. Chest 1994;105:49–52.

PATIENT 55

A 22-year-old man with hemoptysis

A 22-year-old man presented with hemoptysis. Previously in good health, the patient first noted a cough 3 weeks before admission that was initially blood streaked but rapidly progressed to frank hemoptysis. On the day of admission, he estimated that he coughed up 300 ml of "pure blood."

Physical Examination: Vital signs: normal. General: anxious without dyspnea. Head: normal. Chest: crackles in the right mid- and upper-lung fields. Heart: normal heart sounds, without murmurs. Abdomen: normal. Extremities: normal.

Laboratory Findings: Hct 38%, WBC 3,600/μl. Coagulation profile, electrolytes, liver function tests: normal. ABG (room air): pH 7.43, $PaCO_2$ 35 mmHg, PaO_2 88 mmHg. Chest radiograph: right upper and left lower lung field infiltrates.

Questions: What is the differential diagnosis of this patient's hemoptysis? How should he be evaluated?

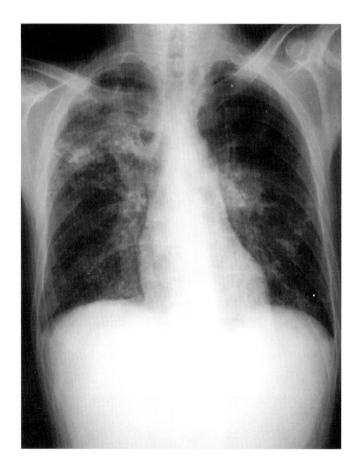

Diagnosis: Active pulmonary tuberculosis with hemoptysis.

Discussion: The sudden onset of hemoptysis in a previously healthy patient is an anxiety-provoking event for both patient and physician. Massive hemoptysis, which is variably defined as 100–600 ml of hemoptysized blood within 12–24 hours, greatly increases a physician's concern because of the potential lethality of this condition. The challenge for managing these patients lies in rapidly identifying the source and etiology of the airway hemorrhage and determining the most effective therapeutic approach.

The differential diagnosis of massive hemoptysis in an individual patient depends on the relative prevalences of different lung diseases within a population. Because these prevalences demonstrate considerable regional variation, the most common conditions associated with hemoptysis vary in different sections of the country. Across the United States, for instance, tuberculosis and bronchiectasis have been traditionally considered to be the most common causes of massive hemoptysis, with lung abscess, lung cancer, intracavitary fungus balls, and mitral stenosis accounting for airway bleeding in a smaller number of patients. In the midwestern United States, however, a recent investigation demonstrated that the incidences of bronchiectasis and active tuberculosis as a cause of hemoptysis are only 1% and 7%, respectively, because these conditions are less prevalent in this region of the country. The major causes of bleeding identified in this study were bronchitis (37%) and bronchogenic carcinoma (19%).

The primary diagnostic approach to patients with hemoptysis focuses on the localization of the bleeding site by bronchoscopy. In patients with massive hemoptysis, rigid bronchoscopy is generally preferred because of its greater ability to suction airway blood compared to the fiberoptic instrument. Recently, however, a prospective study demonstrated that high-resolution chest CT can determine the source and etiology of hemoptysis in 61% of patients compared to the 43% who are diagnosed by fiberoptic bronchoscopy alone. In addition, CT can suggest a diagnosis in 50% of the patients who undergo nondiagnostic bronchoscopic examinations. The final diagnoses in this study included bronchiectasis (25%), tuberculosis (16%), lung cancer (12%), intracavitary fungus ball (12%), and bronchitis (5%). In 19% of cases, the hemoptysis was cryptogenic. These observations indicate that high-resolution chest CT can serve as a useful adjunct to bronchoscopy and may in some instances have a greater diagnostic yield. Although clinically useful, however, CT scanning does not obviate the need for bronchoscopy.

In an effort to determine outcome of patients with significant bleeding, an investigative group in the southeastern United States retrospectively identified 59 consecutive patients who presented with at least 200 ml of blood in a 24-hour period. Only 4 of the 59 patients required surgery and the remainder recovered with medical management alone. In this series, no patient with bronchitis, bronchiectasis, or active tuberculosis as a cause of hemoptysis died during 10 years of follow-up. Risk factors for a poor clinical outcome included a diagnosis of carcinoma, nonoperability, and hemoptysis of greater than 1000 ml of blood during 24 hours.

The present patient underwent a chest CT scan that demonstrated a right upper lobe cavity considered to be the likely source of bleeding and an infiltrate in the lower lobe consistent with aspirated blood. Bronchoscopy detected active bleeding in the posterior segment of the right upper lobe. Lavage samples obtained at bronchoscopy demonstrated acid-fast bacilli. The patient was placed on antituberculous medication and did not require surgery. The hemoptysis resolved and the patient successfully completed the course of chemotherapy.

Clinical Pearls

1. Active tuberculosis and bronchiectasis are important causes of hemoptysis in many regions of United States, particularly in inner cities where tuberculosis is especially prevalent.

2. High-resolution CT scanning of the chest can be an extremely useful adjunct to diagnosis and complements information obtained with fiberoptic bronchoscopy.

3. Major episodes of hemoptysis due to active tuberculosis usually respond to antituberculous therapy without a need for surgical resection.

REFERENCES
1. Corey R, Hla KM. Major and massive hemoptysis: reassessment of conservative management. Am J Med Sci 1987;294:301–309.
2. Johnston H, Reisz G. Changing spectrum of hemoptysis: underlying causes in 148 patients undergoing diagnostic flexible fiberoptic bronchoscopy. Arch Intern Med 1989;149:1666–1668.
3. Jones DK, Davies RJ. Massive haemoptysis: medical management will usually arrest the bleeding. BMJ 1990;300:889–890.
4. McGuiness G, Beacher JR, Harkin TJ, et al. Hemoptysis: prospective high-resolution CT/bronchoscopic correlation. Chest 1994;105:1155–1162.

PATIENT 56

A 43-year-old man with HIV infection and multidrug-resistant tuberculosis

A 43-year-old man with a history of HIV infection and multidrug-resistant tuberculosis presented to the hospital with cough and fever. The patient's tuberculosis was initially diagnosed 3 years earlier after which he sporadically took prescribed antituberculosis drugs. Two years prior to the present admission, he underwent a left lower lobectomy for treatment of hemoptysis. Six months prior to admission, a sputum culture grew *M. tuberculosis* resistant to isoniazid, rifampin, streptomycin, ethambutol, and ethionamide. He was placed on a regimen consisting of multiple second-line drugs, which he took in an irregular manner.

Physical Examination: Temperature 104°F, other vital signs normal. General: ill-appearing man. Head: normal. Neck: shotty bilateral cervical adenopathy. Chest: scattered crackles throughout all lung fields. Heart: normal heart sounds. Abdomen: normal. Extremities: normal. Neurologic: normal.

Laboratory Findings: Hct 33%, WBC 5,600/μl. Na$^+$ 129 mEq/L. Liver function tests: normal. Arterial blood gases (room air): PaO$_2$ 67 mmHg, PaCO$_2$ 30 mmHg, pH 7.53. CD4+ cell count: 250/μl. Chest radiograph: bilateral fibronodular infiltrates with cavitations. Sputum smears: positive for acid-fast organisms.

Questions: How should this patient's multidrug-resistant tuberculosis be treated? What steps should be taken to assure compliance?

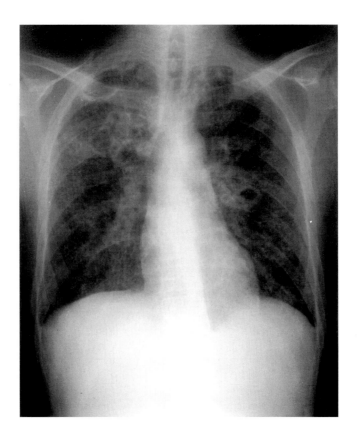

Diagnosis: Multidrug-resistant tuberculosis in a patient with HIV infection.

Discussion: Occasionally patients with tuberculosis present the clinician with seemingly insurmountable problems. The present patient, for instance, has a diffuse pulmonary infection with a strain of *M. tuberculosis* that is resistant to essentially all first-line medications and has underlying AIDS with severe immunosuppression. Previously, such patients had a median survival of 2 months, with essentially no patients surviving to 1 year. Recent observations indicate, however, that a rational and aggressive drug regimen with close patient monitoring can prolong survival beyond what has been previously reported.

Drug selection for patients with tuberculosis should always be guided by the organism's sensitivity pattern with the inclusion of at least two bactericidal drugs. In patients with multidrug-resistant tuberculosis, however, these goals may not be achievable because the limited number of available agents to which the isolate is sensitive. In general, pyrazinamide is usually added to the regimen because it is active and bactericidal only at a pH of 5; therefore, sensitivity testing for this drug is not entirely reliable. Among the remaining drugs that are available for drug-resistant isolates, para-aminosalicylic acid (PAS), cycloserine, kanamycin, and capreomycin have a long record of use in tuberculosis. Newer agents that may be useful in management of patients with multi-drug resistant organisms include ansamycin (rifabutin) and the quinolones. Other newer agents, such as clarithromycin, amoxicillin-clavulanic acid, and clofazimine, will probably have little impact on the management of drug-resistant tuberculosis.

In designing a drug regimen for patients with multi-drug resistant tuberculosis, the first principle is to obtain sensitivity testing for all second-line drugs. Only certain reference laboratories or the Centers for Disease Control perform reliable testing for these agents. Local departments of health are good resources for learning where to send isolates.

Guided by drug sensitivities, adherence to the following principles further assists selection of an effective regimen. Aminoglycosides should be added whenever possible with use of amikacin or kanamycin as first-choice drugs. Neither of these agents typically has cross-resistance with streptomycin. Baseline audiograms must be obtained and renal function should be closely monitored. Capreomycin, a compound related to the aminoglycosides, usually does not demonstrate cross-resistance with amikacin or kanamycin. Capreomycin should not, however, be used in combination with these two aminoglycosides because of additive toxic effects.

A quinolone, such as ofloxacin or ciprofloxacin, is generally added to an aminoglycoside regimen. Quinolones have excellent in vitro activity against *M. tuberculosis* and most, with the exception of sparfloxacin, have good side effect profiles. Clear demonstration of efficacy, however, awaits the completion of large clinical trials. Ofloxacin may have an advantage over ciprofloxacin because MICs for *M. tuberculosis* are generally better for the former agent. Levofloxacin, which consists solely of the l-isomer of ofloxacin (the active form of the drug), has been used but fewer data exist than for ofloxacin and ciprofloxacin regarding its efficacy in tuberculosis. The quinolones should be avoided in pregnancy and used selectively in children because of the sparse safety data and reports of quinolone-induced arthropathy.

In addition to pyrazinamide, an aminoglycoside, and a quinolone, two additional agents are generally added to the regimen. Unfortunately, significant cross-resistance occurs between rifampin and rifabutin, so this agent is unlikely to benefit patients with rifampin-resistant isolates. Both PAS and ethionamide produce frequent gastrointestinal side effects, and it is usually difficult to use both of these drugs in the same patient. Cycloserine is occasionally associated with severe psychiatric effects, including paranoia and suicidal ideation.

After determination of a drug regimen, two other principles of therapy should be considered. First, medications must be administered in a directly observed therapy (DOT) setting. Second, care must be supervised by a physician experienced in the care of multidrug-resistant tuberculosis. Treatment of isoniazid- and rifampin-resistant tuberculosis should be continued for at least 18–24 months.

The present patient was treated with a regimen consisting of ciprofloxacin (750 mg bid), capreomycin (1 gm/day), cycloserine (500 mg bid), pyrazinamide (1.5 gm/day), and PAS (4 gm tid). He was also enrolled in a DOT program, with which he was compliant. He responded to therapy and his sputum converted to negative, but he died 15 months later of another AIDS-related illness.

Clinical Pearls

1. Multidrug-resistant tuberculosis may be assoicated with somewhat longer survival than has generally been reported if a drug regimen is carefully chosen and adminstered.

2. Sensitivity testing against second-line agents is difficult and should be done only by reliable reference laboratories. An injectable agent is generally the cornerstone of an MDR regimen.

3. All patients with multidrug resistant tuberculosis must be enrolled in a program of directly observed therapy.

REFERENCES

1. Fischl MA, Daikos GL, Uttamchandani RB, et al. Clinical presentation and outcome of patients with HIV infection and tuberculosis caused by multiple-drug resistant bacilli. Ann Intern Med 1992;117:184–190.
2. Hong Kong Chest Service/British Medical Research Council. A controlled trial of rifabutin and an uncontrolled study of ofloxacin in the retreatment of patients with pulmonary tuberculosis resistant to isoniazid, streptomycin, and rifampicin. Tuber Lung Dis 1992;73:59–67.
3. Iseman MD. Treatment of multidrug-resistant tuberculosis. N Engl J Med 1993;329:784–791.
4. Park M, Davis AL, Rom WM. Denouement of MDR-TB at Bellevue Hospital. Am J Respir Crit Care Med 1994;149:A104.

PATIENT 57

A 55-year-old man with a bronchopleural fistula following resectional surgery for multidrug-resistant tuberculosis

A 55-year-old man was admitted complaining of dyspnea and right-sided pleuritic chest pain. He had been discharged from the hospital 4 weeks earlier following a right upper lobe resection for multidrug-resistant tuberculosis. The surgery had been uncomplicated, and the postoperative period was uneventful. The patient was discharged home on a regimen of pyrazinamide, ethambutol, streptomycin, ofloxacin, and ethionamide, all of which were to be administered under a program of directly observed therapy.

Physical Examination: Temperature 100.6°F. General: thin male in no acute distress. Head: normal. Chest: diminished breath sounds over entire right chest. Cardiac: normal. Abdomen: no organomegaly. Neurologic: normal.

Laboratory Findings: Hct: 35%, WBC 12,300/µl. Serum electrolytes: normal. Chest radiograph (shown below): multiple air-fluid levels in the right hemithorax.

Questions: What is the likely cause of this patient's dyspnea and radiographic abnormality? How should the patient be managed?

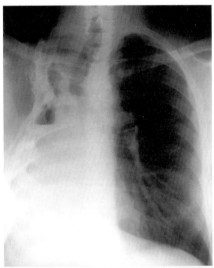

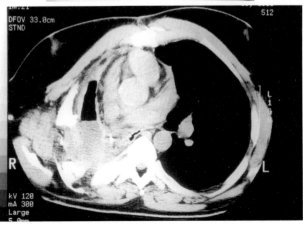

Diagnosis: Bronchopleural fistula complicating lung resection for multidrug-resistant tuberculosis.

Discussion: Multidrug resistant tuberculosis (MDR-TB) has become a common clinical problem in some regions of the United States. In New York City, 11–16% of all patients with tuberculosis have MDR disease. Because of the high lethality of this condition and its poor response to drug therapy, the role of surgical resection of infected lung tissue for the treatment of MDR-TB will become increasingly important. Presently, most clinicians experienced in the care of patients with MDR-TB will consider surgical interventions in any patient who has tuberculosis resistant to both isoniazid and rifampin. Once both of these agents are "lost," the chance for a cure with medical therapy is greatly diminished. As surgical approaches become more widely applied in the management of tuberculosis, clinicians will require an understanding of the varying techniques and potential complications of this form of care.

In the pre-chemotherapeutic era, surgery played a major role in the treatment of tuberculosis, although the range of surgical procedures employed was quite different from those used today. Thoracoplasty, collapse therapy, insertion of foreign bodies into the pleural space (plombage), and creation of chronic draining fistulae (Eloesser flap) were all fairly common. Currently, the most common operation for MDR-TB tuberculosis is pneumonectomy followed in frequency of use by lobectomy. Selection of the surgical procedure depends on the extent of the tuberculous infection and the patient's underlying ventilatory reserve. Because the remaining lung may be diseased in patients undergoing lobectomies and expand poorly to the chest wall, procedures have been devised in which muscle flaps are placed into the pleural space to avoid residual space problems and bronchial stump leaks.

The largest recently published experience concerning surgical treatment for MDR-TB comes from the National Jewish Hospital in Denver. Of 109 patients with MDR-TB seen at that hospital in the 10-year period from 1983 to 1993, 62 underwent resectional surgery, and 59 of the 62 eventually became sputum negative. Negative sputum cultures are not required before surgery for a good outcome. In the resected group, there was only one bronchopleural fistula and one operative death. There were three late nonsurgical deaths.

Complications of resectional surgery for tuberculosis include hemothorax, atelectasis, pneumonia, and bronchopleural fistulae due to breakdown of the bronchial stump. Of these, the last is the most feared. Breakdown of the bronchial stump usually results from a poor blood supply to the site or to the presence of residual infection. The presence of a bronchopleural fistula typically produces fever and radiographic evidence of an intrapleural air-fluid level. To decrease the incidence of postoperative bronchopleural fistulae, the patient's airways should be evaluated before surgery to determine that the planned site for the stump is free of infection. CT scanning can aid in this determination.

The management of an established bronchopleural fistula presents a difficult clinical challenge. Nonsurgical interventions such as the application of tissue glue may close the fistula and avoid the need for surgery. Most patients, however, require further surgical interventions. Available procedures include insertion of a muscle flap to close the stump, thoracoplasty to eliminate the residual pleural space, and chronic open pleural drainage. Surgical approaches are commonly limited by patients' poor general health and limited ventilatory reserve.

The present patient was initially treated with broad-spectrum antibiotics to manage the intrapleural infection that universally accompanies a bronchopleural fistula. His fever persisted, however, and the chest radiograph did not improve. The patient underwent a thoracoplasty with creation of a muscle flap to cover the bronchial stump. He stabilized and gradually improved, experiencing enhanced control of his MDR-TB.

Clinical Pearls

1. Surgical therapy should be considered in patients with MDR-TB who have a poor response or unfavorable prognosis with medical therapy alone.

2. Selection of patients for resectional surgery should be based on the location and extent of the disease, ventilatory reserve, and the ability of the surgeon to leave uninfected surgical margins around the bronchial stump.

3. Late complications of resection surgery can be avoided by careful selection of patients. The development of postoperative intrapleural air-fluid levels or an increasing pleural effusion indicates the presence of a bronchopleural fistula.

REFERENCES

1. Iseman MD, Madsen L, Goble M, Pomerantz M. Surgical intervention in the treatment of pulmonary disease caused by drug-resistant *Mycobacterium tuberculosis*. Am Rev Respir Dis 1990;141:623–625.
2. Pomerantz M, Madsen L, Goble M, Iseman M. Surgical management of resistant mycobacterial tuberculosis and other mycobacterial pulmonary infections. Ann Thorac Surg 1991;52:1108–1111.
3. Etienne TJ, Spiliopoulos A, Megevand R. Surgery for lung tuberculosis and related lesions: change in clinical presentation as a consequence of migration of population. Acta Chir Belg 1994;94:101–104.
4. Iseman M, Madsen L, Iseman M, Ackerson L. Impact of surgery on the management of MDR-TB. Am J Resp Crit Care Med 1995;151:A336.

PATIENT 58

A 22-year-old woman with chronic abdominal pain and a positive tuberculin skin test

A 22-year-old woman presented with a 6-week history of a dull pain in her lower abdomen. She denied fever, changes in bowel habits, or decreased appetite. The patient had immigrated to the United States four months earlier from Bangladesh where she had been known to have a positive tuberculin skin test. Her physicians had recommended isoniazid prophylaxis, but the patient refused because of her abdominal pain.

Physical Examination: Vital signs: normal. General: comfortable, well-nourished. Lymph nodes: normal. Chest: clear. Cardiac: normal heart sounds without gallops, murmurs or rubs. Abdomen: moderate tenderness in the right lower quadrant with voluntary guarding without rebound, no discrete masses, no organomegaly. Pelvic: normal. Extremities: normal.

Laboratory Findings: CBC, electrolytes, liver function tests: normal. Tuberculin skin test: 16 mm induration. Chest radiograph: normal. HIV antibody: negative: Stool examination: negative for ova, parasites, and acid-fast bacilli. CT scan of abdomen: shown below.

Questions: What is the likely diagnosis? How should the patient be managed?

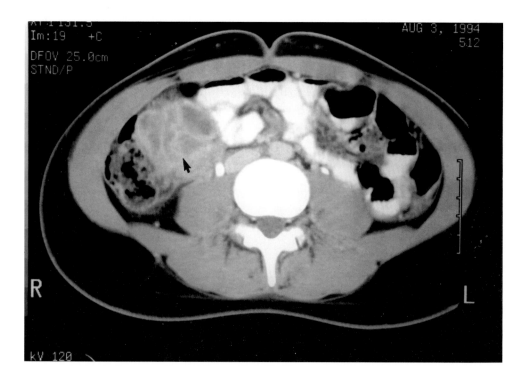

Diagnosis: Ileocecal tuberculosis.

Discussion: Extrapulmonary tuberculosis accounts for approximately 15% of all cases of tuberculosis in the non-AIDS population within the United States. Among those with extrapulmonary disease, peritoneal and gastrointestinal tuberculosis accounts for less than 10% of cases. Peritoneal and gastrointestinal tuberculosis, however, occurs more commonly—as do all forms of extrapulmonary tuberculosis—in patients with AIDS.

Tuberculosis of the gastrointestinal tract is believed to develop by several possible mechanisms: swallowing of infected sputum (probably the most common), consumption of infected milk (unusual in countries where milk is routinely pasteurized), hematogenous spread, and contiguous spread from an infected organ. Several series have emphasized that approximately 80% of patients with gastrointestinal tuberculosis do not have simultaneous active pulmonary tuberculosis. Although abdominal tuberculosis may occur throughout the gastrointestinal tract, the most common site is the ileocecal area. Patients typically present with abdominal pain, weight loss, and fever; less commonly, there may be diarrhea, nausea, vomiting, melena, or rectal bleeding, or the presentation may mimic acute appendicitis. Most patients will have abdominal tenderness, although fewer (< 25%) will have a discrete mass, or "doughy" abdomen, signifying peritoneal inflammation. In cases not treated promptly, obstruction, perforation, and fistula formation may occur.

The initial diagnosis usually considered in patients who present with clinical manifestations of gastrointestinal tuberculosis is Crohn's disease. Of historical interest, before the description of Crohn's disease as a definite clinical entity in 1932, many cases of granulomatous enteritis were misclassified as tuberculosis. The diagnosis of gastrointestinal tuberculosis can be proved definitively only by culturing mycobacteria from a biopsy specimen or by demonstrating improvement after treatment with antituberculous chemotherapy. However, noninvasive studies, primarily gastrointestinal series and abdominal CT scanning, can provide clues to the diagnosis, although the findings can mimic those of Crohn's disease. Barium contrast studies may demonstrate thickening of the ileocecal valve, mucosal irregularities, and contraction and irritation of the cecum. Abdominal CT findings in patients with ileocecal tuberculosis commonly show circumferential wall thickening and thickening of the ileocecal valve, exophytic extension engulfing the terminal ileum, and massive lymphadenopathy with central hypodensity consistent with necrosis. The latter findings, consistent with more severe inflammation and disease, have been noted more often in patients with AIDS. The definitive diagnosis, which requires histopathologic examination and culture of biopsy material, can usually be accomplished at colonoscopy, but may require more invasive approaches. Stool cultures will not reliably grow mycobacteria.

The therapy of ileocecal tuberculosis is no different from that for other forms of extrapulmonary tuberculosis. Many experts advocate empiric therapy in patients from areas that are endemic for tuberculosis if characteristic clinical and radiographic findings are present. Others favor attempting to obtain culture material, because the increasing incidence of drug-resistant tuberculosis makes empiric therapy a less attractive option. Without obtaining pathologic material, one cannot reliably attribute a lack of response to treatment to drug resistance on the one hand or an incorrect diagnosis on the other.

In the present patient, a percutaneous biopsy of the lymph nodes surrounding the ileocecal valve (arrow) was done to obtain material for culture, and the patient was placed on antituberculous therapy. Material obtained from the biopsy did not grow mycobacteria. However, after starting therapy with isoniazid, rifampin, ethambutol, and pyrazinamide, the patient experienced resolution of symptoms within 1 month. A presumptive diagnosis of ileocecal tuberculosis was made. Follow-up abdominal CT scan revealed marked improvement in the lymphadenopathy surrounding the cecum. Treatment was continued for 6 months.

Clinical Pearls

1. Gastrointestinal tuberculosis should be considered in the differential diagnosis of patients with subacute or chronic abdominal pain who have a positive tuberculin test and/or who come from areas endemic for tuberculosis.

2. Findings on abdominal CT may strongly suggest the diagnosis of ileocecal tuberculosis, particularly in advanced cases.

3. Although empiric therapy may be indicated in select cases, it is advisable to obtain material for culture because of the increased incidence of drug-resistant tuberculosis.

REFERENCES

1. Balthazar EJ, Gordon R, Hulnick D. Ileocecal tuberculosis: CT and radiologic evaluation. AJR 1990;154:499–503.
2. Fitzgerald JM, Menzies RI, Elwood RK. Abdominal tuberculosis: a critical review. Dig Dis 1991;9:269–281.
3. Estill MR. Ileocecal tuberculosis in an Asian male immigrant: case report and a literature review. Mt Sinai J Med 1992;59:366–370.
4. Jayanthi V, Probert CS, Sher KS, et al. The renaissance of abdominal tuberculosis. Dig Dis 1993;11:36–44.
5. Marshall JB. Tuberculosis of the gastrointestinal tract and peritoneum. Am J Gastroenterol 1993;88:989–999.

PATIENT 59

A 76-year-old woman with a history of tuberculosis and hemoptysis

A 76-year-old woman presented to the hospital with hemoptysis. The patient had tuberculosis 30 years earlier that was treated for 1 year with a variety of medications that she did not recollect. She had been well until 2 weeks before admission when she developed cough without fever. Two days before admission she began to cough small amounts of bright red blood. Her medical history was notable for hypertension and adult-onset diabetes mellitus.

Physical Examination: Vital signs: normal. General: no acute distress. Head: normal. Chest: crackles in right upper lung field. Heart: normal heart sounds, regular rhythm, without murmurs; Abdomen: normal. Extremities: normal. Neurologic: normal.

Laboratory Findings: Hct 36%, WBC 4,800/μl. Electrolytes and prothrombin time: normal. ABG (room air): pH 7.38, $PaCO_2$ 38 mmHg, PaO_2 90 mmHg. Chest radiograph: cavitary lesion in the left upper lobe. The patient was scheduled for bronchoscopy to evaluate the source of bleeding.

Question: What precautions should bronchoscopists take to reduce their risk of contracting tuberculosis?

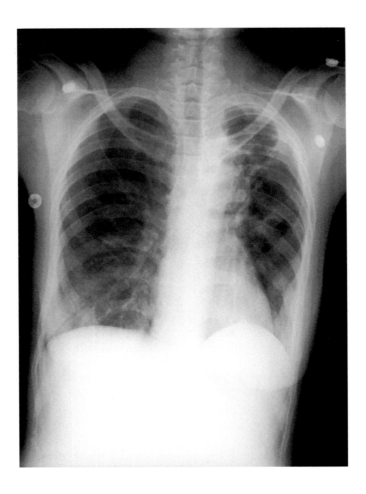

Diagnosis: Hemoptysis due to bronchiectasis in a patient with prior inactive tuberculosis.

Discussion: Major issues in the care of patients with suspected tuberculosis are the problems of nosocomial transmission and the risk of occupational exposure of physicians, nurses, respiratory therapists and others involved in the care of such patients. In the pre-antibiotic era, the risk of developing tuberculosis as an occupational infection was enormous. Several studies, including classic studies involving student nurses, indicated that nearly all health care workers caring for patients with tuberculosis could expect to become infected. A classic early study from the pre-antibiotic era determined that 100% of 227 tuberculin-negative nursing students developed infection over a period of 4 years. The only means available to curb transmission at that time were opening windows and instructing patients to turn away from health care workers when coughing.

In the modern era, reliable statistics on the rate of tuberculosis infection and the clinical settings associated with the greatest risk have been difficult to obtain. It seems likely, however, that activities involving the generation of droplet nuclei (cough-inducing procedures such as bronchoscopy or administration of aerosol pentamidine) will be associated with a high risk of nosocomial transmission of tuberculosis. Indeed, a recent study at a large academic medical center in the United States reported that 86 (24.5%) of 351 physicians were tuberculin positive. Although only 25 (8.6%) of the physicians were definitely known to have been recent tuberculin converters, these data indicate that occupational exposure to tuberculosis in certain health care settings remains a considerable risk. However, recent observations in physician and nonphysician employees working at Barnes Hospital in St. Louis indicate that exposure to tuberculosis in an employee's home community poses a greater risk for tuberculin conversion than exposure on the job in the hospital.

In an effort to assess the occupational risk of pulmonary physicians for acquiring tuberculosis infection, one group used a questionnaire to determine the tuberculin status of pulmonary fellows. By canvassing fellows in 25 cities with the highest rates of tuberculosis in the country, and using the same questionnaire in a control group of infectious disease fellows, they determined that 11% of pulmonary fellows had become infected during their training, whereas only 2.4% of infectious disease trainees had converted their tuberculin skin tests. Although the limitations of such as study are obvious, the authors felt that exposure to cough-inducing procedures such as bronchoscopy likely accounted for the difference in infection rates. (Alternatively, one might conclude that infectious disease fellows do not get close to patients or that pulmonary fellows know nothing about infection control.) A study in Japan attempted to assess the risk among the high-risk groups of pathologists and pathology technicians. They found that pathologists performing autopsies had an odds ratio that ranged between 6 and 10 of tuberculosis infection.

What can be done to reduce the risk of occupational transmission of tuberculosis to bronchoscopists? First and most important is to avoid unnecessary bronchoscopies. When the procedure must be done, as in the case of a patient whose hemoptysis requires investigation and localization, environmental controls assume the greatest importance. Some hospitals have designed their bronchoscopy suites to provide a ventilation efficiency of greater than six air exchanges per hour through high efficiency (HEPA) filters. In addition, ultraviolet lights can kill bacteria in droplet nuclei, with efficacy equivalent to several more air exchanges per hour. Finally, during bronchoscopy, physicians can use particulate respirator masks that contain HEPA filters as well. These measures are in accordance with recent OSHA and CDC regulations. Although the efficacy of these measures in combination have not been demonstrated, it seems reasonable to apply them selectively in areas of the hospital where tuberculosis exposure is expected to be high. The cost of these preventive measures is considerable, and a recent analysis suggests that in areas where tuberculosis is uncommon, a hospital might have to spend in excess of a million dollars to prevent even one case of active tuberculosis.

The present patient underwent bronchoscopy with the environmental controls described above in place. Bleeding was confined to the right upper lobe, and a CT scan of the chest demonstrated bronchiectasis in the same location. All specimens from the bronchoscopy were negative for acid-fast organisms, and the patient was treated with a course of antibacterials, which resolved the hemoptysis.

Clinical Pearls

1. Tuberculosis is a major occupational risk to healthcare workers and should be considered with other issues of safety in the workplace.

2. The best method for reducing occupational transmission of tuberculosis from high-risk procedures is to avoid the procedure. Interventions that induce coughing, such as bronchoscopy, should be applied to patients with known or suspected tuberculosis only when no alternative approaches exist to a diagnosis.

3. Environmental controls are more important than personal respiratory protection; bronchoscopy suites should meet current standards of environmental safety.

REFERENCES

1. Israel HL, Hetherington HW, Ord JG. A study of tuberculosis among students of nursing. JAMA 1941;117:839–844.
2. Nardell EA. Dodging droplet nuclei. Reducing the probability of nosocomial tuberculosis transmission in the AIDS era. Am Rev Respir Dis 1990;142:501–503.
3. Malasky C, Jordan T, Potulski F, Reichman LB. Occupational tuberculosis infections among pulmonary physicians in training. Am Rev Respir Dis 1990;142:505–507.
4. Fraser VJ, Kilo CM, Bailey TC, et al. Screening of physicians for tuberculosis. Infect Control Hosp Epidemiol 1994;15:95–100.
5. Adal KA, Anglim AM, Palumbo CL, et al. The use of high-efficiency particulate air-filter respirators to protect hospital workers from tuberculosis: a cost-effectiveness analysis. N Engl J Med 1994;331:169–173.
6. Centers for Disease Control and Prevention. Guidelines for preventing transmission of *Mycobacterium tuberculosis* in health care facilities, 1994. MMWR 1994;43(RR-13):1–132.
7. Menzies D, Fanning A, Yuan L, Fitzgerald M. Tuberculosis among health care workers. N Engl J Med 1995;332:92–98.
8. Bailey, TC, Fraser VJ, Spitznagel EL, Dunagan WC. Risk factors for a positive tuberculin skin test among employees of an urban, midwestern teaching hospital. Ann Intern Med 1995;122:580–585.

PATIENT 60

A 38-year-old woman with hyperuricemia during treatment for tuberculosis

A 38-year-old woman undergoing drug therapy for pulmonary tuberculosis was noted to have hyperuricemia. She first presented 2 months earlier with a history of cough, night sweats, a 15-pound weight loss, and a chest radiograph suggestive of tuberculosis. Sputum cultures were positive for drug-sensitive *M. tuberculosis,* and she was started on isoniazid 300 mg, rifampin 600 mg, pyrazinamide 1.5 g, and ethambutol 900 mg. Two weeks later, her symptoms improved and her sputum smears converted to negative. The patient had previously had unprotected sex with different partners. Her serum uric acid had been normal at the outset of antituberculous therapy.

Physical Examination: Vital signs: normal. General: chronically ill-appearing woman. Skin: mild seborrheic dermatitis on face. Chest: normal. Abdomen: normal. Lymph nodes: "shotty" lymphadenopathy in cervical, axillary, and inguinal areas. Neurologic: normal.

Laboratory Findings: Hct 34%, WBC 3,200/μl. Electrolytes, renal indices, and liver function tests: normal. Uric acid: 14.5 mg/dl. Sputum: negative for acid-fast bacilli. Chest radiograph: shown below. HIV test: positive. CD4+ cell count: 624/μl.

Question: How should this patient's drug therapy be managed now that 2 months of treatment has been completed?

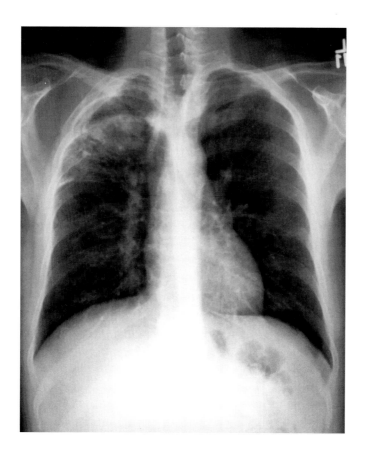

Diagnosis: Pulmonary tuberculosis and pyrazinamide-induced hyperuricemia in a patient with AIDS.

Discussion: Pyrazinamide was first used in the treatment of tuberculosis during the 1950s. Although it was found to be quite effective even for patients with organisms resistant to isoniazid and streptomycin, it fell out of use because of an unacceptable rate of hepatotoxicity. Hepatotoxicity is dose-related, however, and occurs in as many as 15% of patients treated with 50 mg/kg of the drug, which was the standard dosage used in the 1950s. When used at the currently recommended dose of 15–25 mg/kg, pyrazinamide does not seem to increase the risk of liver injury in regimens that include isoniazid and rifampin compared to the risk of these two drugs used without pyrazinamide. Therefore the use of pyrazinamide does not change the recommendations for hepatotoxicity monitoring that should be employed for isoniazid and rifampin.

Hyperuricemia almost always occurs in patients treated with pyrazinamide. Because gout or other complications of hyperuricemia rarely develop, monitoring of uric acid levels is not necessary during the course of treatment with pyrazinamide. A baseline measurement of serum uric acid before initiating treatment, however, may aid in identifying pyrazinamide as the etiologic factor if gout does develop during therapy. Arthralgias that are not consistently associated with elevated uric acid levels may also be seen. These symptoms can usually be controlled with non-steroidal anti-inflammatory agents. Photosensitivity with skin discoloration may also occur, as may gastrointestinal intolerance unrelated to liver injury. Rare hypersensitivity reactions have been reported.

Ethambutol is the best tolerated of the antituberculous medications. The most common adverse effect is retrobulbar neuritis, usually manifested by decreased visual acuity, central scotomata, and red-green color blindness. This toxicity is dose-related: it occurs in less than 1% of patients given a daily dose of 15 mg/kg, and in about 5% of patients receiving 25 mg/kg daily. The lower dose is recommended for patients on daily therapy without evidence of drug-resistant tuberculosis, and the low incidence of toxicity does not warrant periodic ophthalmologic exams during therapy. The higher dose, which may be bactericidal, is recommended when treating drug-resistant tuberculosis that is susceptible to ethambutol; these patients should probably have a baseline exam of visual acuity and red-green discrimination. All patients taking ethambutol should be instructed to report any visual problems. This side effect almost always reverses upon stopping the drug. There is greater concern for this complication in two groups: patients with renal insufficiency and children too young for visual acuity testing. As ethambutol is renally excreted, renal impairment causes increased serum levels leading to increased toxicity. Dosage adjustment is required in these patients, and ocular screening is advisable. Ethambutol should be used with caution in young children, and perhaps avoided if other agents are acceptable alternatives. Other side effects are rare, and include rash, hyperuricemia, and gout.

Antituberculous therapy has been reported to cause a higher incidence of adverse effects in patients with HIV infection, with reported rates ranging from 4–18%. The complications with increased rates include skin rash, gastrointestinal disturbances, and liver injury. Some authors have noted the difficulty in accurately ascribing toxicities in these patients to the treatment for tuberculosis, due to the variety of other explanations for complications: most patients are on other potentially toxic medications, the liver or skin may be involved with tuberculosis or another infection, or HIV itself may be the culprit. When therapy for tuberculosis does seem to cause toxicity, the implicated drug is almost always isoniazid or rifampin. More cautious monitoring for hepatotoxicity may be warranted in AIDS patients receiving these medications. At this point in our experience, there seems to be no reason for increased concern in using pyrazinamide or ethambutol in AIDS patients.

The present patient was compliant with her treatment in a directly observed therapy program. The presence of hyperuricemia in the absence of gout did not require alteration of her drug therapy. Because the patient had completed 2 months of therapy for a drug sensitive strain, pyrazinamide and ethambutol were stopped. She completed a 6-month course of therapy with isoniazid and rifampin.

Clinical Pearls

1. At currently used doses, pyraizinamide does not seem to increase the risk of hepatotoxicity when added to isoniazid and rifampin.

2. Pyrazinamide so commonly increases the serum uric acid level that the presence of this finding is a positive indicator that patients are taking their medications. Pyrazinamide-induced hyperuricemia, however, rarely causes clinical gout.

3. The most common side effect of ethambutol is retrobulbar neuritis, which is dose-related and reversible.

4. All patients given ethambutol should be warned to report visual problems such as decreased visual acuity or red-green color blindness, but baseline exams are probably needed only in patients taking daily doses of 25 mg/kg, and periodic exams are not recommended.

5. Ethambutol should be used with caution in patients with renal insufficiency and children too young for visual exams; alternative therapies should be considered in these patients.

REFERENCES

1. Somner AR, Brace AA. Ethionamide, pyrazinamide, and cycloserine used successfully in the treatment of chronic pulmonary tuberculosis. Tubercle 1962;43:345–360.
2. Perez-Stable EJ, Hopewell PC. Current tuberculosis treatment regimens: choosing the right one for your patient. Clin Chest Med 1989;10:323–339.
3. American Thoracic Society. Treatment of tuberculosis and tuberculosis infection in adults and children. Am J Respir Crit Care Med 1994;149:1359–1374.
4. Jones BE, Otaya M, Antoniskis D, et al. A prospective evaluation of antituberculous therapy in patients with human immunodeficiency virus infection. Am J Respir Crit Care Med 1994;150:1499–1502.

PATIENT 61

A 28-year-old man with HIV infection and persistently positive sputum cultures on therapy for tuberculosis

A 28-year-old man with HIV infection presented with cough and fever. The patient was diagnosed with pulmonary tuberculosis 7 months earlier when a sputum culture grew pan-sensitive *M. tuberculosis*. He had been placed initially on a self-administered drug regimen of isoniazid, rifampin, pyrazinamide, and ethambutol, but continued to have symptoms for several months. Present medications included isoniazid, rifampin, zidovudine, haloperidol, and folic acid.

Physical Examination: Temperature 101°F, other vital signs normal. General: chronically ill-appearing man. Head: normal. Neck: shotty cervical adenopathy. Chest: left upper lung field crackles. Heart: normal heart sounds, without murmurs; Abdomen: normal. Neurologic: normal.

Laboratory Findings: Hct 32%, WBC 7,900/μl. Liver function tests: normal. Chest radiograph: right apical and left lower lung zone infiltrates. Sputum examination: numerous acid-fast bacilli.

Questions: Why are the patient's sputum smears positive so long into therapy? What is appropriate management at this point?

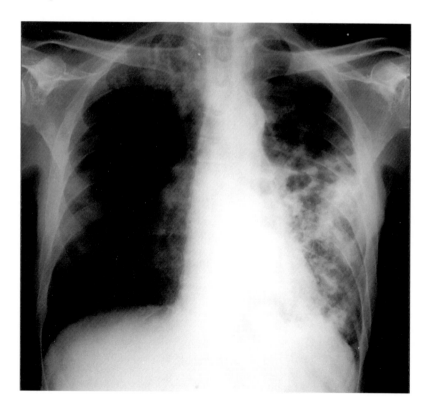

Diagnosis: Failure of drug therapy for pan-sensitive tuberculosis in a patient with AIDS.

Discussion: Persistence of symptoms and positive acid-fast smears in a patient who is on a drug regimen that should be effective presents a difficult clinical problem. Indeed, the regimen of isoniazid, rifampin, pyrazinamide, and ethambutol for 2 months followed by 4 more months of isoniazid and rifampin is one of the so-called "100% effective" regimens of the modern chemotherapy era. Treatment failures (failure to sterilize the sputum during treatment) should be exceedingly rare, and relapse rates (recurrence of smear-positive disease after completion of therapy) with this regimen should be less than 3.5%. In addition, the initial burden of mycobacteria (extent of radiographic abnormalities, or the number of acid-fast bacteria seen on sputum examination) should generally not affect the response or cure rate. Thus, what should a clinician do when faced with apparent failure of an effective drug regimen?

The initial approach is to assess the relatively few reasons for treatment failure. The most obvious and most common is failure of patients to take their medications. The realization of the magnitude of the problem of noncompliance has led to the widespread institution of directly observed therapy (DOT) programs and strong public health recommendations to enroll as many patients as possible in them. Because tuberculosis represents a public health hazard, the onus is on the physician, rather than the patient, to ensure compliance.

A second consideration in apparent drug failure is drug-resistant tuberculosis. Given the increasing incidence of drug-resistant tuberculosis in the United States, drug-susceptibility testing should be performed on all initial isolates. If no appreciable clinical response occurs after 3–6 months of therapy, susceptibility testing should be repeated to guarantee that sensitivity patterns have not changed as a result of erratic self-administration of drugs. Sensitivity testing should be done in a reliable and experienced reference laboratory whenever there is a question of drug resistance.

Two other more complex causes of drug failure are both related to HIV infection. Although studies have indicated that effective chemotherapy regimens should achieve bacteriologic cure with high frequency in HIV-infected patients, several investigations have demonstrated accelerated mortality in patients coinfected with HIV and tuberculosis. The reason for this observation may be that tuberculosis appears to accelerate the progression of HIV disease, and the host immune system becomes completely depleted. In this regard, immunomodulating therapies, such as thalidomide or γ-interferon (recently shown to have some benefit in selected patients with HIV infection and disseminated *M. avium* infections), may one day prove useful in tuberculosis.

Finally, malabsorption of drugs may be another reason for treatment failure in patients with HIV infection. Several patients with AIDS have been reported who appeared to be failing treatment but in fact were being inadequately treated because of low blood levels of antituberculous medications. In an AIDS patient with diarrhea or other evidence of malabsorption who does not appear to be responding to appropriate therapy, serum levels of antituberculous medications should be obtained to guide drug dosing. Drug levels need not be obtained routinely, however, because they have never been shown to affect outcome in tuberculosis, and therapeutic ranges for antituberculous medications have not been well established. Drug levels should be performed only by experienced reference laboratories.

The isolate obtained from the present patient 7 months after the start of therapy was still sensitive to all antituberculous medications. The patient admitted to poor compliance with therapy. He was enrolled in a DOT program and demonstrated rapid improvement in symptoms and clearing of sputum cultures.

Clinical Pearls

1. Noncompliance with therapy remains the most common reason for failure of apparently adequate treatment regimens.

2. Sensitivity testing should be performed by competent laboratories in all cases of apparent treatment failures.

3. Malabsorption of drugs should be considered as a cause of treatment failure in AIDS patients who have a history of diarrhea.

REFERENCES

1. Peloquin CA, MacPhee AA, Berning SE. Malabsorption of antimycobacterial medications. N Engl J Med 1993;329:1122–1123.
2. Gordeon SM, Horsburgh CR, Peloquin CA, et al. Low serum levels of oral antimycobacterial agents in patients with disseminated *Mycobacterium avium* complex disease. J Infect Dis 1993;168:1559.
3. Wallis RS, Vjecha M, Amir-Tahmasseb M, et al. Influence of tuberculosis on human immunodeficiency virus (HIV-1): enhanced cytokine expression and elevated β2-microglobulin in HIV-1-associated tuberculosis. J Infect Dis 1993;167:43–8.

PATIENT 62

A 68-year-old man with a remote history of tuberculosis and a productive cough

A 68-year-old man presented with recurrent bouts of purulent, blood-streaked sputum most recently occurring during the past 2 weeks. He reported a history of pulmonary tuberculosis 40 years earlier while living in China. He had been treated with iatrogenic pneumothorax for about 1 year. He subsequently had received medical therapy with an unknown pill combined with an intramuscular drug injection for more than 1 year. In the ensuing years he had experienced pneumonia in the treated lung several times and often required antibiotics for prolonged courses. He currently denied fever, chills, night sweats, weight loss, and chest pain. He admitted dyspnea on climbing three flights of stairs.

Physical Examination: Temperature 99.8°F. Chest: decreased breath sounds throughout left side, particularly at the base. Remainder of examination normal except for the presence of clubbing.

Laboratory Findings: WBC 8,400/μl, differential normal. Electrolytes: normal. Chest radiograph and CT scan: shown below.

Question: What is the nature of the left-sided radiographic changes?

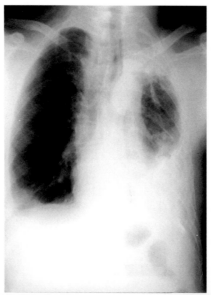

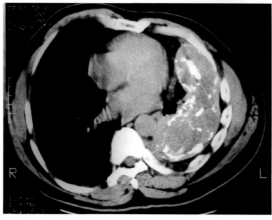

Diagnosis: Fibrothorax with calcification.

Discussion: Fibrothorax is a term commonly used to describe the thick, fibrous peel that remains adherent to the visceral pleura after the resolution of an intense inflammatory process. Tuberculosis follows hemothrax and empyema as the leading causes of fibrothorax; other conditions less commonly complicated by fibrothorax include pancreatitis, collagen-vascular-related pleural disease, asbestos pleurisy, and uremia. Patients who underwent repeated therapeutic pneumothoraces as treatment for pulmonary tuberculosis in the pre-chemotherapeutic era often developed fibrothorax as a complication, and such patients may occasionally still be seen.

With time, the fibrous tissue encasing the lung contracts, reducing the volume of the hemithorax and the underlying lung. This causes an ipsilateral mediastinal shift and decreased mobility of the lung. Functionally, this results in a restrictive defect, which rarely may be severe enough to cause ventilatory failure. Imbalance between the reductions in ventilation and perfusion to the trapped lung may ensue, with the perfusion significantly more affected.

The radiographic appearance of fibrothorax is that of chronic pleural thickening that can lead to a progressively smaller lung volume over months to years. The layer closest to the lung frequently calcifies; this serves as a marker of chronicity and can be used to measure the thickness of the peel.

In addition to ventilatory problems, posttuberculosis fibrothorax also may be complicated by occurrence of a bronchopleural fistula (BPF). In a series of 15 patients with tuberculosis-related BPF, 7 had a fibrothorax prior to presentation. Only 2 of the 7 patients had active tuberculosis at the time of the BPF; 3 patients (2 with fibrothorax due to therapeutic pneumothoraces and 1 with prior tuberculous pleurisy) had had a fibrothorax present for over 30 years before the BPF occurred. The contribution of a rigid pleura unable to seal a leak, as well as the perfusion impairment in the lung parenchyma, to the development of the BPF remains speculative.

Treatment of fibrothorax with surgical decortication should be reserved for patients whose restrictive defect causes persistent or progressive symptoms, as some patients who have posttuberculous pleural thickening may have spontaneous resolution over several months. Decortication involves stripping the thickened peel from the visceral pleura. If a cleavage plane between the peel and the visceral pleura cannot be established, serious morbidity from multiple persistent air leaks can follow. With successful procedures, the vital capacity can improve as much as 50%, if the underlying lung parenchyma is relatively healthy. Significant improvement of dyspnea after decortication has been reported in a patient whose fibrothorax had been present for 44 years.

The present patient developed a bacterial lung abscess in the left lower lobe days after presentation, with poor response to parenteral antibiotics. Fluid from the abscess cavity subsequently spilled throughout the tracheobronchial tree, and the patient died of respiratory failure.

Clinical Pearls

1. The thick peel of fibrous tissue adherent to the visceral pleura that is the residua of an inflammatory pleuritis is called a fibrothorax.
2. Hemothorax, empyema, and tuberculosis are the most common causes of fibrothorax.
3. Fibrothorax may be complicated by restrictive physiology or bronchopleural fistulae.
4. Decortication of fibrothorax may relieve dyspnea and improve vital capacity up to 50% even decades after the peel has formed.

REFERENCES
1. Donath J, Khan FA. Tuberculous and posttuberculous bronchopleural fistula. Chest 1984;86:697–703.
2. Light RW. Fibrothorax. In: Light RW, ed. Pleural Diseases, 2nd ed. Philadelphia: Lea & Febiger, 1995, pp 291–292.
3. Deslauriers J, Perrault LP. Fibrothorax and decortication. Ann Thorac Surg 1994;58:267–268.

PATIENT 63

A 69-year-old woman with bilateral lung nodules and seizures

A 69-year-old woman was admitted complaining of a chronic cough, fever, weight loss, and generalized weakness. The cough was productive of white sputum. The past medical history was notable for hypothyroidism, for which she was taking synthroid, and an episode of multilobar pneumonia 10 years earlier.

Physical Examination: Temperature 101.2°F, pulse 88, respirations 18, blood pressure 110/70. General: thin, chronically ill-appearing woman. Skin: dry. Head: normal. Chest: coarse breath sounds throughout. Heart: normal. Abdomen: normal. Extremities: normal.

Laboratory Findings: Hct 34%, WBC 25,000/μl. Electrolytes and liver function tests: normal. Arterial blood gas (room air): pH 7.46, PCO_2 37 mmHg, PO_2 54 mmHg. Tuberculin skin test and anergy panel: no reactions. Sputum Gram stain: mixed flora. Sputum AFB smear: negative. Chest radiograph: multiple nodular densities in both lungs with areas of confluence.

Hospital Course: The patient underwent a fiberoptic bronchoscopy and transbronchial biopsy. Twenty-four hours after bronchoscopy, the patient had a generalized seizure, and a head CT scan revealed multiple nodular lesions with surrounding areas of edema. Biopsy of the lesions revealed organisms that were weakly acid-fast, and silver-stain-positive.

Questions: What is the diagnosis? What therapy should be instituted?

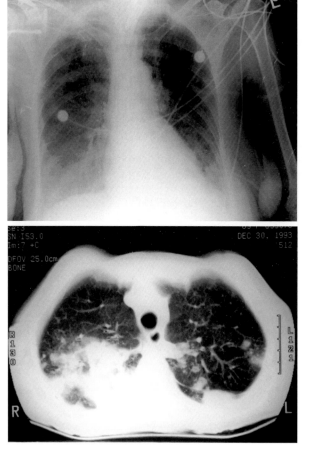

Diagnosis: Nocardiosis.

Discussion: Nocardia species are gram-positive, soil-dwelling organisms that are rare causes of disease in humans. Because nocardiosis occurs primarily in patients with altered immune defenses, the incidence of this disorder is increasing as more patients in recent decades are being treated with intensive chemotherapeutic regimens and undergoing immunosuppressive therapy for organ transplantation. Patients with lymphoreticular malignancies and those treated with corticosteroids are at particular risk. Patients with advanced AIDS have more recently been reported to be subject to nocardia infections. It should be noted, however, that some patient series report that up to one-half of patients have no identifiable immunodeficiency. Also, nocardia also appears capable of "colonizing" the upper airway without acting as a pathogen.

Nocardia asteroides is the species that most commonly causes disease, although infections caused by *brasiliensis* and *transvalensis* have also been reported. Infection occurs by inhalation, and the lungs are involved in approximately 80% of patients with nocardiosis. Disseminated disease is common, with noncutaneous extrapulmonary disease occurring in over 80% of patients with profound immune dysfunction. Approximately one-quarter of patients will have central nervous system (CNS) involvement, usually a brain abscess, which denotes a poor prognosis. Cutaneous disease in the form of multiple skin abscesses is a common manifestation.

Patients without CNS disease typically present with a 1–6 month history of nonspecific symptoms such as fever, weight loss, and cough. Those with CNS involvement tend to have a less indolent presentation, often with duration of symptoms as short as 1 week presenting with headaches or seizures. Chest radiographs are usually abnormal in all forms of nocardiosis, with single or multiple lobar infiltrates, nodules, abscesses, adenopathy, and pleural effusions all described. The radiographic appearance often suggests tuberculosis. Further complicating diagnosis, up to one-quarter of patients with AIDS and nocardial lung infections may have a previous history of or concurrent mycobacterial infections.

The diagnosis of nocardiosis is usually made by finding in respiratory secretions characteristic branching, filamentous, gram-positive rods that are also weakly acid-fast. Morphologic recognition is important in making a rapid diagnosis, as cultures may take as long as 4 weeks for growth to appear. Therefore, routine bacterial cultures may miss the diagnosis unless the laboratory is alerted to hold the samples longer than the customary 48–72 hours; growth of nocardia species on fungal or mycobacterial cultures often provides the first suggestion of the disease when the diagnosis is not suspected. Most commonly a rapid diagnosis is made by identification of the organism in histologic specimens (e.g., transbronchial or brain biopsy specimens) against a background of suppurative, nongranulomatous inflammation, or in material drained from abscesses.

Because the clinical manifestations of nocardiosis are nonspecific or may simulate other disorders, such as tuberculosis, seriously ill patients may not be appropriately treated in a timely fashion and die of their disease. Unfortunately, the initial diagnosis is often made postmortem from autopsy specimens. Even with early diaganosis and the prompt initiation of appropriate therapy, mortality in patients with CNS nocardiosis approaches 50%. The majority of patients with isolated pulmonary disease respond to therapy, although this form still has a 10% mortality.

With the exception of extrapulmonary abscesses, which usually need drainage, treatment for nocardiosis is primarily medical. The sulfonamides remain the mainstay of therapy; minocycline, amikacin, erythromycin, and imipenem are acceptable alternatives. The utility of susceptibility testing is not entirely clear, although some authors recommend their routine use to guide antibiotic selection. While in vitro testing has suggested synergy of certain drug combinations, e.g., trimethoprim-sulfamethoxazole or erythromycin-ampicillin, improved clinical efficacy of drug combinations over single-drug therapy has not been demonstrated. Treatment for a prolonged duration is necessary; 6 months seems to be the minimum, and as much as 12 months may be necessary in the setting of CNS disease or AIDS.

The current patient's brain biopsy grew *Nocardia asteroides,* confirming the diagnosis of pulmonary nocardiosis with CNS involvement. He was treated for 12 months with sulfamethoxazole, with a good clinical response.

Clinical Pearls

1. Nocardia is an unusual pathogen that typically affects patients who have conditions that depress cell-mediated immunity, such as malnutrition, AIDS, or corticosteroid therapy.

2. The clinical presentation and chest radiographic appearance of nocardiosis may simulate tuberculosis; both diseases may be present concurrently in patients with AIDS.

3. Patients with nocardiosis often have disseminated disease. CNS involvement with a brain abscess portends a poor clinical course.

4. Nocardiosis requires prolonged treatment for at least 6–12 months to effect a cure.

REFERENCES

1. Bross JE. Gordon G. Nocardial meningitis: case reports and review. Rev Infect Dis 1991;13:160–165.
2. Javaly K, Horowitz HW, Wormser GP. Nocardiosis in patients with human immunodeficiency virus infection: report of 2 cases and review of the literature. Mediane 1992;71:128–138.
3. Conant EF, Wechsler RJ. Actinomycosis and nocardiosis of the lung. J Thorac Imag 1992;7:75–84.

PATIENT 64

A 50-year-old man with diabetes mellitus and a pleural effusion

A 50-year-old man was admitted to the hospital complaining of 4 days of fever, chills, and a productive cough. Three years earlier, he was noted to have a positive tuberculin skin test, but isoniazid preventive therapy was not prescribed. His past medical history was notable for longstanding insulin-dependent diabetes mellitus and a remote history of intravenous drug use.

Physical Examination: Temperature 101°F. General: comfortable. Chest: dullness to percussion and diminished breath sounds at the right base.

Laboratory Findings: Hct 28%, WBC 5,000/ul. Electrolytes, liver function tests, coagulation profile: normal. HIV antibody: negative. Chest radiograph: left lower lobe infiltrate and pleural effusion.

Questions: What is the cause of the pleural effusion? How should the patient be treated?

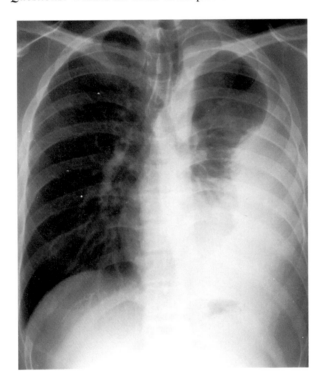

Pleural fluid analysis

Appearance: serous

Nucleated cells: 3850/µl

Differential: 75% lymphocytes

Total protein: 3.7 gm/dl

LDH: 210 IU/L

Glucose: 65 mg/dl

pH: 7.32

AFB smear: negative

Diagnosis: Tuberculous pleurisy in a diabetic patient.

Discussion: Diabetes mellitus is a recognized risk factor for developing active tuberculosis in patients with positive tuberculin skin tests. Although the exact nature of the immune defect in diabetes that predisposes to active tuberculosis is unclear, investigators have postulated a link between the two diseases. In a series of 1,250 patients followed over a 7-year period in Africa, 5% developed pulmonary tuberculosis. Three-quarters of the cases of tuberculosis developed coincident with or after the onset of clinical diabetes; the prevalence of tuberculosis was greater in insulin-dependent than in non–insulin-dependent diabetes. The mortality from tuberculosis in this group of patients was 24%, which is an extremely high rate in the chemotherapy era.

In a second report by the same investigators examining a separate cohort of patients, the prevalence of glucose intolerance among patients with tuberculosis was found to be at least four times higher in patients with tuberculosis than in the general population. This finding provides further evidence for a link between diabetes and tuberculosis.

The impact of diabetes on the clinical presentation and course of tuberculosis has been studied by Japanese and American investigators. Using CT scans of the chest, the Japanese compared the radiographic findings of tuberculosis in 31 patients with diabetes and 71 patients with no underlying disease. The diabetic patients had a higher incidence of a nonsegmental distribution of infiltrates (30% vs. 3%, p<0.01) and multiple small cavities within a single lesion (44% vs. 5%, p<0.01). The likelihood of finding an atypical localization of pulmonary infiltrates—in either the basal segments of the lower lobes, the anterior segment of the upper lobes, or the right middle lobe—was not different between groups. In a smaller retrospective series from the United States no difference in the incidence of multilobar involvement was found between diabetic and nondiabetic patients with tuberculosis.

No differences exist in the drug therapy for tuberculosis in patients with or without underlying diabetes. Rare reports exist, however, of an increased insulin requirement in patients treated with rifampin. Because hyperglycemia can interfere with host phagocytic cell function, blood glucose should be tightly controlled in diabetic patients with tuberculosis, as is the case with any infection. Physicians should be reminded of the inclusion of diabetes mellitus in the group of underlying illnesses that predispose a patient with a positive tuberculin skin test to the development of active tuberculosis. Had the present patient received isoniazid preventive therapy according to the ATS guidelines, he would not have developed tuberculous pleurisy.

The present patient's lymphocyte-predominant exudative pleural effusion in the setting of underlying diabetes and a positive tuberculin skin test were strongly suggestive of the diagnosis of tuberculous pleurisy. A pleural biopsy confirmed the diagnosis by showing necrotizing granulomas. A reminder was sent to the patient's primary physician to consider more seriously isoniazid preventive therapy for patients with diabetes and a positive tuberculin skin test.

Clinical Pearls

1. Diabetes mellitus increases the chance of developing active tuberculosis in patients with latent infection and should be included in the risk / benefit evaluation when considering isoniazid preventive therapy.

2. Although data are inconclusive, diabetics with tuberculosis may present with atypical radiographic findings. Clinicians should maintain a high index of suspicion for tuberculosis when evaluating pulmonary syndromes in these patients.

3. Treatment of tuberculosis in diabetic patients is no different than in nondiabetic patients, although serum glucose and insulin dosage should be closely monitored during therapy.

REFERENCES

1. Root, HF. The association of diabetes and tuberculosis. N Engl J Med 1934;210:1–13.
2. Swai AB, McLarty DG, Mugusi F. Tuberculosis in diabetic patients in Tanzania. Trop Doct 1990;20:147–150.
3. Mugusi F, Swai AB, Alberti KG, McLarty DG. Increased prevalence of diabetes mellitus in patients with pulmonary tuberculosis in Tanzania. Tubercle 1990;71:271–276.
4. Ikezoe J, Takeuchi N, Johkoh T, et al. CT appearance of pulmonary tuberculosis in diabetic and immunocompromised patients: comparison with patients who had no underlying disease. AJR 1992;159:1175–1179.
5. Morris JT, Seaworth BJ, McAllister CK. Pulmonary tuberculosis in diabetics. Chest 1992;102:539–541.

PATIENT 65

A 36-year-old HIV-positive woman with fever, weight loss, and an abnormal chest radiograph

A 36-year-old woman with advanced AIDS was admitted with fever and weight loss of 5 weeks' duration. She had a dry cough but denied shortness of breath or chest pain. The patient had a previous history of *Pneumocystis* pneumonia and took prophylactic trimethoprim-sulfamethoxazole.

Physical Examination: Temperature 102.3°F, pulse 82, respirations 18, blood pressure 110/70. General: thin, ill-appearing. Head: temporal wasting. Chest: scattered rhonchi throughout. Cardiac: no murmurs. Abdomen: no organomegaly. Extremities: thin and wasted. Neurologic: alert and oriented.

Laboratory Findings: Hct 29%, WBC 2,700/μl. Serum electrolytes, liver function tests: normal. Chest radiograph (shown below): right upper lobe cavitary infiltrate. Sputum AFB stain: positive. CD4+ cell count: 10/μl.

Clinical Course: The patient was started on isoniazid, rifampin, pyrazinamide, and ethambutol for a presumptive diagnosis of pulmonary tuberculosis. Subsequently, blood cultures grew *M. avium–intracellulare*.

Questions: What was the cause of the patient's abnormal chest radiograph and positive sputum AFB smear? What therapy should be instituted?

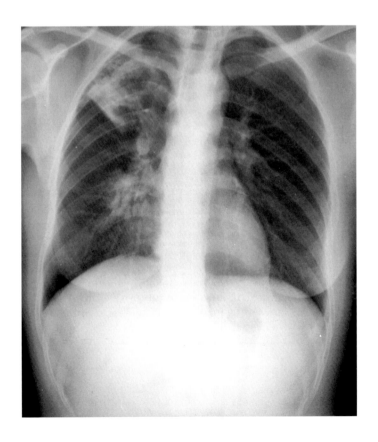

Diagnosis: Pulmonary tuberculosis and disseminated infection with *M. avium-intracellulare* in a patient with advanced AIDS.

Discussion: Infections with organisms from the *M. avium* complex (MAC) are a major cause of morbidity and mortality in patients with HIV infection. Before the AIDS epidemic, disseminated MAC infections were exceedingly rare. Presently, this infection remains primarily confined to patients with HIV disease. Indeed, as patients with HIV infection are living longer as a result of prophylaxis against many of the major AIDS-related pathogens, such as *Pneumocystis carinii,* disseminated MAC infections are becoming increasingly common.

Unlike *M. tuberculosis, M. avium* causes disease through progression of a primary infection rather than the reactivation of latent infection. The cardinal manifestations of the disease are fever and weight loss in patients with a CD4+ count <100 cells/μl. The chest radiograph, however, in patients with AIDS complicated by disseminated MAC infections is usually normal. Less than 5% of patients have focal radiographic abnormalities. Radiographic abnormalities typical of pulmonary tuberculosis in a patient with AIDS should prompt the exclusion of that disease even in the presence of an established MAC infection.

The finding of a positive sputum smear for acid-fast bacilli, even in the AIDS era, is still strongly suggestive of tuberculosis. A recent patient series from the San Francisco General Hospital reported that the positive predictive value for pulmonary tuberculosis of an expectorated sputum sample that was stain positive for acid-fast organisms was 87% in a group of patients with and without HIV disease. The positive predictive value of a positive acid-fast smear of a sputum that was collected by induction or a bronchoalveolar lavage specimen was 70% and 71%, respectively. These predictive values did not differ between patients with and without HIV disease. A positive sputum acid-fast smear, therefore, should always strongly suggest the diagnosis of pulmonary tuberculosis regardless of the clinical setting.

It may be difficult to confirm the diagnosis of pulmonary tuberculosis, however, in AIDS patients who have concomitant disseminated MAC infections. Although pulmonary parenchymal abnormalities in these patients result from infection with *M. tuberculosis,* sputum samples may also harbor MAC organisms from airway colonization. Because MAC bacilli are "rapid growers," they may overgrow and conceal the presence of *M. tuberculosis* in culture specimens, thereby obscuring the diagnosis of pulmonary tuberculosis.

Distinguishing between *M. tuberculosis* and MAC disease is important because of the different therapeutic approaches. Although the optimal therapy for MAC infections in patients with AIDS has yet to be determined, most regimens currently employ a macrolide antibiotic (usually clarithromycin in a dose of 500 mg b.i.d.), a rifamycin (such as rifabutin), and ethambutol. Of these, only ethambutol has reliable activity against *M. tuberculosis.* The resistance and sensitivity patterns for any individual strain of *M. tuberculosis* may differ for rifabutin and rifampin, and rifabutin sensitivity testing of *M. tuberculosis* is not routinely done in most laboratories. A regimen consisting solely of clarithromycin, rifabutin, and ethambutol, therefore, would be expected to have low efficacy in treating tuberculosis.

It is important to exclude the presence of tuberculosis in patients being considered for prophylaxis against MAC infection. Current guidelines recommend the initiation of rifabutin preventive therapy when a patient with AIDS has a CD4+ count < 100/μl. If the patient harbors *M. tuberculosis,* however, single drug prophylactic therapy with rifabutin presents a substantial risk for the emergence of rifampin-resistant tuberculosis because of the cross-resistance patterns of these two agents. Resistance to rifampin represents a considerable barrier to developing an effective drug regimen that will result in an effective cure. Because patients with AIDS often have subtle or atypical radiographic manifestations of tuberculosis, a high index of suspicion must be maintained. If there is any question regarding the presence of tuberculosis, rifabutin prophylaxis should be withheld until after a thorough diagnostic evaluation.

The present patient had radiographic features highly suggestive of pulmonary tuberculosis. Repeated sputum cultures, however, failed to demonstrate *M. tuberculosis* because the cultures were overgrown with *M. avium-intracellulare.* Nevertheless, she was treated for both tuberculosis and disseminated MAC disease with isoniazid, rifampin, pyrazinamide, ethambutol, and clarithromycin. She expired 3 weeks later with unresponsive disease. An autopsy isolated *M. tuberculosis* from her lungs.

Clinical Pearls

1. Although disseminated disease from *M. avium* complex organisms occurs commonly in patients with HIV infection, focal pulmonary disease due to these pathogens rarely occurs. Patients may have concomitant MAC and *M. tuberculosis* infections.

2. A positive acid-fast smear in a patient with AIDS and an abnormal chest radiograph is more likely to represent pulmonary tuberculosis than MAC disease.

3. Before instituting rifabutin prophylaxis in patients with advanced HIV infection, pulmonary tuberculosis should be rigorously excluded, particularly in patients with abnormal chest radiographs or respiratory symptoms.

REFERENCES

1. Tenholder MF, Moser RJ, Tellis CJ. Mycobacteria other than tuberculosis. Pulmonary invovlement in patients with acquired immunodeficiency syndrome. Arch Intern Med 1988;148:953–955.
2. Nightingale SD, Cameron DW, Gordin FM. Two controlled trials of rifabutin prophylaxis against *Mycobacterium avium* complex infection in AIDS. N Engl J Med 1993;329:828–834.
3. Yajko DM, Nassos PS, Sanders CA, et al. High predictive value of the acid-fast smear for *Mycobacterium tuberculosis* despite the high prevalence of *Mycobacterium avium* complex in respiratory specimens. Clin Infect Dis 1994;19:334–336.
4. Rigsby MO, Curtis AM. Pulmonary disease from nontuberculous mycobacteria in patients with human immunodeficiency virus. Chest 1994;106:913–919.

PATIENT 66

A 52-year-old man with tuberculosis and a pneumothorax

A 52-year-old man presented with chest pain and dyspnea 3 days after discharge from the hospital where he had been started on therapy for pulmonary tuberculosis. He had been diagnosed with pulmonary tuberculosis 6 weeks earlier on the basis of an abnormal chest radiograph and sputum smears positive for acid-fast bacilli. Sputum cultures subsequently grew *M. tuberculosis,* and the patient's sputum smears converted to negative on a regimen of isoniazid, rifampin, pyrazinamide, and ethambutol. Sensitivities subsequently revealed that the organism was resistant to isoniazid and streptomycin.

Physical Examination: Temperature 99°F, respirations 26, pulse 90, blood pressure 130/76. General: thin, moderate respiratory distress. Chest: absent breath sounds over the right chest. The remainder of the examination was normal.

Laboratory Findings: CBC normal. Na^+ 119 mEq/L. Liver function tests: normal. ABG (room air): pH 7.37, PCO_2 30 mmHg, PO_2 72 mmHg. Chest radiograph: absence of lung markings in the right chest with an air fluid level.

Questions: What is the diagnosis? What should be the initial management?

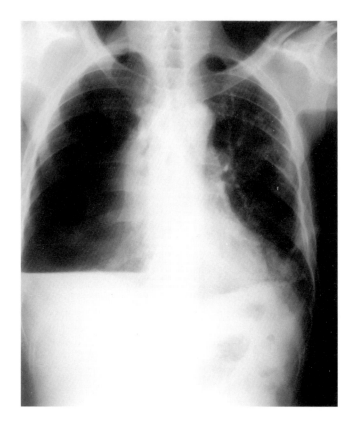

Diagnosis: Bronchopleural fistula (BPF) in a patient with active pulmonary tuberculosis.

Discussion: The absence of lung markings combined with an air-fluid level are radiographic findings that are diagnostic for a hydropneumothorax. The absence of prior surgery or instrumentation of the chest in the present patient indicates that a spontaneous BPF from active pulmonary tuberculosis has occurred. The development of BPF is one of the most serious and problematic complications of pulmonary tuberculosis and is associated with considerable morbidity and mortality. Although in the modern chemotherapy era, the incidence of BPF formation is considerably less than previously reported, it still presents a formidable management problem to pulmonologist and surgeon.

In current practice, tuberculosis is a relatively rare cause of BFP. Most BPFs result from breakdown of a surgical stump after operation for lung resection or lung transplant. This complication occurs after 2–13% of such operations, and the fistulae may develop hours to years following the procedure. Predisposing factors include infection and/or ischemia at the site of the resection. Advances in surgical technique have decreased the incidence of postoperative BPF. BPFs in the setting of necrotizing bacterial pneumonia or the adult respiratory distress syndrome in patients on mechanical ventilation are relatively common.

The development of a BPF in a patient with tuberculosis is a result of destruction of lung tissue by chronic necrotizing infection. In an older review of BPFs conducted over a 13-year period, it was found that 23 of 77 of fistulae developed spontaneously in patients treated for pulmonary tuberculosis. Virtually all the rest occurred in patients who had undergone resectional surgery (most of these surgeries were for tuberculosis).

Patients with a BPF usually present acutely with dyspnea and chest pain, but can present in a subacute or chronic manner with persistent fevers and weight loss. The typical radiographic features quickly indicate the presence of a BPF.

The morbidity and mortality of patients with BPF are substantial. In a large series of 77 patients, only 57% could be definitively cured, and the overall mortality rate was 20%. In the patients who developed spontaneous BPF, 13 of 23 had positive sputum cultures for *M. tuberculosis* at the time the BPF developed.

Although the diagnosis of BPF is generally straightforward, therapy can often be problematic. An experienced surgeon should always be involved in the patient's management. Initial therapy centers on establishing early surgical drainage with tube thoracostomy, even if an empyema is not present. If there is a delay in pleural space drainage, chronic tuberculous empyema and possibly calcific pleuritis may develop, which will lead to obliteration of the pleural space and loss of pulmonary function. Although tube drainage sometimes leads to lung reexpansion and closure of the fistula, the typical patient will require more definitive therapy. In lieu of surgery, less invasive attempts at definitive therapy can be attempted using tissue adhesive or fibrin glue or an absorbable gelatin sponge (Gelfoam) through the bronchoscope. Experience with these bronchoscopic techniques is largely anecdotal, making their success rate difficult to judge.

The choice of the surgical procedure requires good judgment based on extensive clinical experience with this condition because several different surgical options are available. The primary goal of surgery is to achieve permanent closure of the fistula; however, in some patients palliation is the only realistic expectation. Surgical options include thoracoplasty, extrapleural pneumonectomy, decortication, simple pneumonectomy, or window thoracostomy (Eloesser flap). The choice of operation is based primarily on the condition of the pleural space and the amount of disease in the affected lung. Chest CT and bronchoscopy with the instillation of contrast (fistulogram) will provide useful information in evaluation of the lung and pleural space. When the lung and pleural space have been severely damaged so that a surgical procedure cannot be performed, chronic tube drainage may be the only alternative. There have been reports of patients treated with chronic tube drainage surviving for years.

The present patient had a chest tube inserted with reexpansion of the lung; however, there was a persistent air leak and failure of closure of the BPF. One month after development of the BPF, the patient had a successful decortication and abrasion.

Clinical Pearls

1. Development of an air-fluid level in the pleural space of a patient with active tuberculosis signals a bronchopleural fistula and/or tuberculous empyema.

2. Immediate tube drainage of the pleural space is always indicated to prevent chronic tuberculous empyema and destruction of the pleural space.

3. The morbidity and mortality of BPF from active tuberculosis are substantial, and most patients require a surgical attempt at closure of the fistula.

REFERENCES

1. Hankins JR, Miller JE, Attar S, et al. Bronchopleural fistula: thirteen-year experience with 77 cases. J Thorac Cardiovasc Surg 1978;76:755–762.
2. Hulnick DH, Naidich DP, McCauley DI. Pleural tuberculosis evaluated by computed tomography. Radiology 1983;149:759–765.
3. Donath J, Khan FA. Tuberculous and post-tuberculous bronchopleural fistula: ten-year clinical experience. Chest 1984;86: 697–703.
4. Powner DJ, Bierman MI. Thoracic and extrathoracic bronchial fistulas. Chest 1991;100:480–486.

PATIENT 67

A 36-year-old man with a painful testicular mass

A 36-year-old man presented with complaints of fever, chills, and right testicular pain. He had been seen previously at another hospital where a PPD skin test was reportedly positive. The patient had been a prisoner and was an intravenous drug user.

Physical Examination: Temperature 100°F, other vital signs normal. General: thin, ill-appearing. Head: normal. Chest: scattered crackles, more pronounced at the right apex. Heart: normal heart sounds, without gallops, murmurs, or rubs. Abdomen: normal. Genitalia: fluctuant, tender right testicular mass. Extremities: normal. Neurologic: normal.

Laboratory Findings: CBC and electrolytes: normal. Chest radiograph (shown below): normal. HIV antibody: positive. Testicular biopsy: granulomata with acid-fast organisms.

Questions: What is the pathogenesis of the testicular process in this patient? How should it be treated?

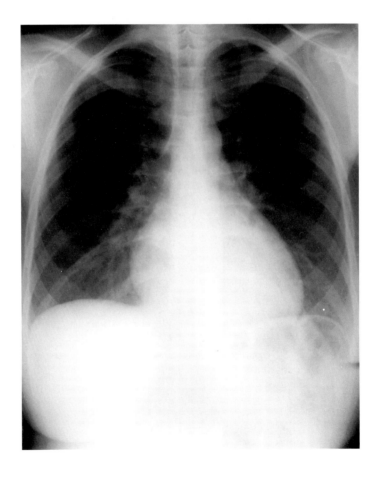

Diagnosis: Tuberculous epididymo-orchitis (disseminated tuberculosis).

Discussion: Genitourinary tuberculosis is a well-known complication of tuberculosis, and usually results from reactivation of a focus of infection in the kidneys that has been dormant for many years. In one of the largest and most classic series, Christensen reviewed 102 cases of genitourinary disease and found a long lag time in most patients between the initial infection and the development of genitourinary disease. In other older reviews, it has been noted that lesions are usually found in both kidneys upon pathologic examination despite the absence of clinical evidence of bilateral disease. This observation supports the concept that genitourinary tuberculosis represents disseminated disease.

The symptoms and signs of genitourinary disease include fever, flank pain, pyuria, and hematuria. As with pulmonary tuberculosis, symptoms may be insidious, and considerable destruction of renal tissue may occur before a diagnosis is made. Although acid-fast organisms may on occasion be demonstrated by direct examination of urine, the triad of an abnormal chest radiograph (seen in 50–75% of cases), a positive tuberculin skin test, and repeatedly sterile pyuria strongly suggests the diagnosis.

Isolated genital tuberculosis occurs less commonly, and represents approximately 10–15% of genitourinary tract disease. Christensen reported that 14 of 102 patients had isolated epididymo-orchitis, and noted that most of these patients did not have pulmonary symptoms. The mechanism of disease in these patients is most likely related to dissemination from an original pulmonary focus. A recent case report, however, suggests that tuberculous epididymitis may occur from sexual intercourse with a partner who has pelvic tuberculosis. This observation raises the possibility of female-to-male venereal transmission. Similarly, acid-fast organisms have been recovered from semen in men with genitourinary tuberculosis, suggesting that male-to-female transmission may also occur.

Traditionally, diagnosis of tuberculosis epididymitis has been made by excisional or open biopsy with demonstration of granulomas and acid-fast organisms. Recently, however, the use of fine-needle aspiration and sonographic examination has opened the way to a less invasive diagnostic approach. In a recent study, notable sonographic findings in 12 cases of tuberculous epididymitis included an enlarged epididymis, predominantly in the tail region, and marked heterogeneity of the echo texture of the involved epididymis. When there is associated testicular involvement, typical sonographic findings include a diffusely enlarged hypoechoic testis, ill-defined focal intratesticular hypoechoic areas, or an irregular margin between the testis and epididymis. These findings may allow differentiation of tuberculous disease from nontuberculous epididymitis. Of note, sonographic studies of patients with genital tuberculosis find a high incidence of asymptomatic renal, ureteral, and bladder lesions. Less than 10% of patients with genital tuberculosis have a positive urine culture for mycobacteria, and only 20% have an abnormal chest radiograph.

The treatment of genitourinary tuberculosis is the same as for pulmonary disease. Most patients will have a good response to medical management with little need for excisional surgery except in exceptional cases where symptoms persist despite therapy. The present patient was treated initially with a four-drug regimen. After cultures revealed that his disease was caused by a pan-sensitive strain of *M. tuberculosis,* isoniazid and rifampin were continued for a total of 6 months of therapy, with excellent clinical results. The patient's chest radiograph remained normal throughout the course of therapy.

Clinical Pearls

1. Epididymitis in the setting of an abnormal chest radiograph and a positive tuberculin skin test should raise the possibility of tuberculous epididymitis.

2. Scrotal sonography can provide strong evidence for tuberculous infection if findings of an enlarged epididymal tail and heterogeneity of the echo texture of the involved epididymis are seen.

3. Fine-needle aspiration is often sufficient for diagnosis and can obviate the need for orchiectomy in most patients.

REFERENCES

1. Christensen WI. Genitourinary tuberculosis: review of 102 cases. Medicine 1974;53:377–390.
2. Wolf JS, McAnich JW. Tuberculous eipididymo-orchitis: diagnosis by fine-needle aspiration. J Urol 1991;145:836–838.
3. Kim SH, Pollack HM, Cho KS, et al. Tuberculous epididymitis and epididymo-orchitis: sonographic findings. J Urol 1993; 150:81–84.

PATIENT 68

A 51-year-old man with hemoptysis and a past history of tuberculosis

A 51-year-old man presented to the hospital with hemoptysis of roughly one cup per day for the preceding week. He had a distant history of treated tuberculosis, and 3 months prior to admission he had a similar episode that resolved with antibacterial therapy. Mycobacterial cultures from that admission were all negative. He denied fever or night sweats, but had lost 5 pounds in the month prior to admission.

Physical Examination: Vital signs: normal. General: comfortable. Head: bitemporal wasting. Chest: coarse rhonchi throughout all lung fields, fine crackles at right base. Cardiac: normal heart sounds, without murmurs, gallops, rubs. Abdomen: without masses, organomegaly. Extremities: normal. Neurologic: normal.

Laboratory Findings: Hct 39%, platelets 316,000/μl, WBC 6,500/μl, prothrombin time 0.5 sec above control. Serum electrolytes: normal. ABG (room air): pH 7.39, PCO_2 33 mmHg, PO_2 78 mmHg. Chest radiograph: scarring and pleural density right upper lobe. Fiberoptic bronchoscopy: no active bleeding, bronchoscopic aspirates negative on smear for acid-fast organisms.

Question: What is the likely etiology of this patient's hemoptysis?

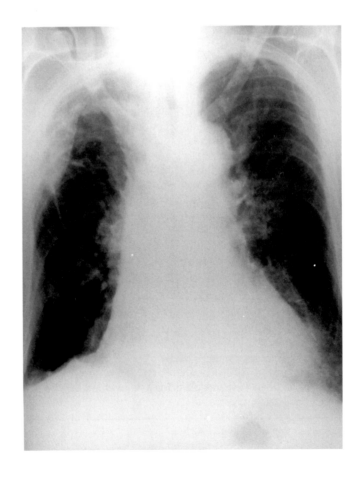

Diagnosis: Hemoptysis due to bronchiectasis caused by tuberculosis (inactive).

Discussion: Common causes of significant or life-threatening hemoptysis include bronchiectasis, tuberculosis, mycetoma, carcinomas, and alveolar hemorrhage. The precise etiology of hemoptysis depends to a certain extent on the demographics of the patient population being studied. Although hemoptysis as a symptom of chest disease is less likely to be due to tuberculosis than other causes, recent literature still suggests that truly massive hemoptysis (variously defined) is often due to tuberculosis in certain settings. One series from South Africa found that 85% of 120 consecutive patients with greater than 200 ml of hemoptysis in 24 hours had a primary diagnosis of tuberculosis. In an Italian series, 31% of 209 patients with hemoptysis severe enough to require bronchial artery embolization had tuberculosis. On the other hand, in the United States, one study from a Veterans Administration hospital reviewed 264 patients who underwent bronchoscopy for the evaluation of hemoptysis (not necessarily massive) and found that tuberculosis was the etiology in only 15 patients (6% of the total), 9 of whom had active disease. However, it should be noted that the patient population at this hospital consisted primarily of older men with smoking histories, in whom cancer (29%) and bronchitis (23%) accounted for the majority of cases of bleeding. The patients in the South African report were generally younger.

Tuberculosis has long been associated with hemoptysis; indeed, this has been one of the most dramatic and often frightening manifestations of the disease since it was initially described centuries ago. Hemoptysis may be a feature of both active tuberculosis as well as a sequela of prior disease, and the mechanisms by which bleeding develops are several. In a recent study of 163 consecutive patients with smear-positive tuberculosis seen in a clinic in Ethiopia, 52% of patients had a presenting complaint of hemoptysis, although the frequency of this sign increased as the total duration of symptoms increased—that is, patients who presented early in the course of tuberculosis were less likely to cough blood than those with advanced disease.

The etiology of bleeding in tuberculosis was set forth by a series of investigators in a classic group of papers that span the introduction of effective antibiotic therapy. Rasmussen's aneurysm, an ectatic blood vessel that traverses a tuberculous cavity where it can be invaded by mycobacteria and exposed to proteases and other inflammatory products that weaken the vessel wall, is perhaps the most feared cause of hemoptysis because the bleeding is often sudden, massive, and fatal. A second cause of hemoptysis in tuberculosis is simple bronchiectasis, whereby there is proliferation of bronchial arteries that form anastomoses with the pulmonary circulation which are vulnerable to erosion by the chronic inflammation characteristic of this disorder. Alternatively, a lymph node may calcify and become a broncholith, which can cause varying degrees of bleeding if the stone erodes through the wall of the airway. Finally, healed and mycobacteriologically sterile cavities may become colonized with fungus, the classic example being the aspergilloma. These mycetomas bleed commonly, and the hemoptysis can be life-threatening.

The importance of considering tuberculosis in the differential diagnosis of hemoptysis is underscored by that fact that nosocomial transmission of the infection often occurs in cases where tuberculosis is unsuspected. Because patients with significant bleeding often undergo procedures that can expose medical personnel to respiratory secretions (bronchoscopy, intubation), failure to consider tuberculosis may lead to transmission of mycobacteria when proper infection control measures are not taken.

The present patient was treated with antibiotics, cough suppressants, and bed rest. Based on CT scan findings that showed ectatic airways in the right upper lobe, his physicians concluded that the bleeding was due to residual bronchiectasis rather than active tuberculosis, and antituberculous medications were not restarted. Subsequently, all mycobacterial cultures were negative. Bleeding did not recur.

Clinical Pearls

1. Tuberculosis remains the most common cause of hemoptysis in many areas of the world. Even in countries where tuberculosis is less common, the disease or its sequelae still account for a significant percentage of bleeding episodes.

2. Hemoptysis is usually a somewhat late symptom in the natural history of tuberculosis, so that prompt recognition and institution of therapy will decrease the chance of serious bleeding.

3. Truly massive hemoptysis, a life-threatening emergency, can be caused by active as well as inactive tuberculosis, and care must be taken to ensure adequate infection control during procedures that increase exposure to respiratory secretions.

REFERENCES

1. Teklu B. Symptoms of pulmonary tuberculosis in consecutive smear-positive cases treated in Ethiopia. Tuber Lung Dis 1993;74:126–128.
2. Cremaschi P, Nascimbene C, Vitulo P, et al: Therapeutic embolization of bronchial artery: a successful treatment in 209 cases of relapse hemoptysis. Angiology 1993;44:295–299.
3. Knott-Craig CJ, Oostuizen JG, Rossouw G, et al: Management and prognosis of massive hemoptysis. Recent experience with 120 patients. J Thorac Cardiovasc Surg 1993;105:394–397.
4. Santiago S, Tobias J, Williams AJ. A reappraisal of the causes of hemoptysis. Arch Intern Med 1991;151:2449–2451.

PATIENT 69

A 59-year-old man with an abnormal chest radiograph and diffuse vesicular skin lesions

A 59-year-old man with insulin-dependent diabetes presented to the hospital complaining of fever and fatigue of 2 weeks' duration. He had noted a 10-pound weight loss in the past month. The patient denied cough, sputum production, and other symptoms.

Physical Examination: Temperature 104°F, respirations 22, pulse 110, blood pressure 140/70. General: ill-appearing. Skin: multiple vesicular lesions on the trunk and extremities. HEENT: normal. Chest: diffuse crackles bilaterally. Cardiac: normal heart sounds without murmurs or rubs. Abdomen: normal. Extremities: normal. Neurologic: normal.

Laboratory Findings: Hct 35.7%, WBC 2,300/μl. Na$^+$ 128 mEq/L, glucose 201mg/dl. ABG (room air): pH 7.40, PCO$_2$ 38 mmHg, PO$_2$ of 70 mmHg. Chest radiograph (shown below): left upper lobe infiltrate. Sputum smear: positive for acid-fast bacilli.

Question: What is the cause of the patient's skin lesions?

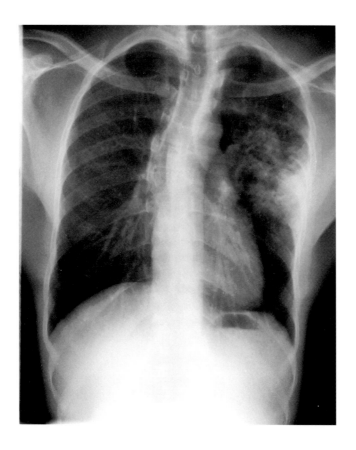

Diagnosis: Tuberculosis cutis miliaris disseminata.

Discussion: The most well known of all cutaneous syndromes related to infection with mycobacteria is undoubtedly leprosy caused by *Mycobacterium leprae.* However, several other mycobacteria, including *Mycobacterium tuberculosis,* can also cause skin disorders.

Cutaneous disease due to *M. tuberculosis* can take several forms that have different pathogenetic mechanisms. First, patients without a previous history of tuberculosis can develop cutaneous disease if they experience direct inoculation of the skin or mucus membranes with mycobacteria. This form of skin disease is termed primary cutaneous tuberculosis due to exogenous infection. A second mechanism occurs by exogenous infection in a patient with a previous history of tuberculosis. These patients can develop an exuberant "wart-like" local reaction at the site of reinfection, resulting in a lesion known as tuberculosis verrucosa cutis. The third mechanism occurs via endogenous hematogenous dissemination. This form of cutaneous disease may result in a variety of conditions, including lupus vulgaris, orificial tuberculosis, a metastatic tuberculous abscess, scrofuloderma, and tuberculosis cutis miliaris disseminata.

Of the cutaneous forms of endogenous hematogenous dissemination, lupus vulgaris is the most common. It represents an immune response in the skin to the organisms. In this condition, reddish lesions distributed over the face and extremities progress slowly over years; the lesions can regress after therapy.

Tuberculosis cutis miliaris disseminata is a manifestation of miliary tuberculosis with cutaneous involvement. A diffuse erythematous papular eruption develops followed by tiny vesicles that first rupture and then crust over, leaving a small scar. There are typically 20–30 of these lesions distributed in a random pattern. The histopathology of the lesions demonstrates an inflammatory infiltrate composed primarily of lymphocytes and neutrophils, usually with focal necrosis. Granulomas are not often seen. Acid-fast bacilli can usually be demonstrated in the biopsy material, and cultures are most often positive.

A fourth form of cutaneous tuberculosis is known as tuberculids. These eruptions are immunologically mediated lesions that develop in patients with pulmonary tuberculosis. Although it is generally impossible to recover organisms by culture of these lesions, recent experiments with the polymerase chain reaction have demonstrated the presence of DNA of *M. tuberculosis* in affected skin tissue. The load of organisms in these lesions is undoubtedly small, which explains why culture results are negative. This form of cutaneous tuberculosis also responds to antituberculous therapy.

The differential diagnosis of the immunologically mediated forms of cutaneous tuberculosis includes sarcoidosis, leprosy, swimming-pool granuloma caused by *M. marinum,* sporotrichosis, and chromomycosis, which is a deep fungal infection caused by organisms belonging to the genus *Phialophora.*

Recently, cutaneous tuberculosis has been reported as a manifestation of disseminated disease in patients with AIDS. Presumably, this disorder is yet another demonstration of the impact of profound underlying immunosuppression on the natural history of tuberculosis.

The present patient underwent skin biopsy that demonstrated acid-fast bacilli without granulomas in the tissue samples. These samples subsequently grew *M. tuberculosis.* The appearance of the lesions and the patient's clinical presentation were consistent with the diagnosis of tuberculosis cutis miliaris disseminata. He was treated with a standard antituberculous regimen, and the skin lesions resolved.

Clinical Pearls

1. Skin disease due to tuberculosis can be caused by direct inoculation of immune or nonimmune hosts, hematogenous dissemination of organisms, or by immune reactions in patients with localized disease.

2. Tuberculosis cutis miliaris disseminata is an unusual manifestation of disseminated tuberculosis. Smears and cultures of affected tissue are usually positive for *M. tuberculosis.*

3. Cutaneous manifestations of tuberculosis should respond to standard antituberculous chemotherapy if the patient is infected with drug-susceptible organisms.

REFERENCES

1. Rohatgi PK, Palazzolo JV, Saini NB. Acute miliary tuberculosis in acquired immunodeficiency syndrome. J Am Acad Dermatol 1992;26:356–359.
2. Victor T, Jordaan HF, Van Nierkerk DJ, et al. Papulonecrotic tuberculid. Identification of *Mycobacterium tuberculosis* DNA by polymerase chain reaction. Am J Dermatopathol 1992;14:491–495.
3. Sehgal VN, Bhattacharya SN, Jain S, et al. Cutaneous tuberculosis: the evolving scenario. Int J Dermatol 1994;33:97–104.

PATIENT 70

A 32-year-old woman with AIDS, a prior history of treated tuberculosis, fever, and cough

A 32-year-old woman with AIDS presented with several months of fever, dyspnea, and a cough productive of white sputum. She had a history of tuberculosis 6 years earlier that had been treated with "several drugs" for 9 months. The patient also had a history of pneumonia due to *Pneumocystis carinii*.

Physical Examination: Temperature 104°F, pulse 110, respirations 25, blood pressure 100/70. General: thin, ill-appearing woman in moderate distress. Head: normal. Neck: shotty cervical adenopathy. Throat: oral thrush. Chest: coarse crackles in both upper lung fields. Abdomen: normal. Neurologic: normal

Laboratory Findings: Hct 21%, WBC 4,100/µl. Electrolytes, liver function tests, coagulation profile: normal. CD4+ cell count: 156/µl. Chest radiograph (shown below): bilateral upper lobe cavities. Chest radiograph (2 years before admission): normal.

Question: Consider the likelihood that this patient's illness is tuberculosis. What would be the pathogenesis of the pulmonary disorder?

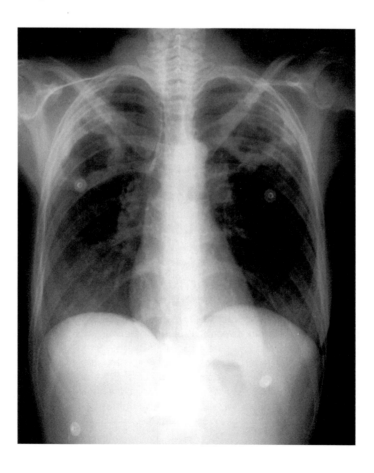

Diagnosis: Tuberculosis in a patient with AIDS most likely due to reinfection with mycobacteria.

Discussion: Respiratory disorders remain a major source of morbidity and mortality for patients with AIDS. Although the differential diagnosis of radiographic abnormalities is extensive in this clinical setting, bacterial pneumonia, pulmonary tuberculosis, and *Pneumocystis* pneumonia are the leading diagnoses in patients with AIDS who present with a new pulmonary infiltrate. In patients with advanced AIDS and severe immunocompromise, deep fungal infections, such as aspergillosis, coccidioidomycosis, and cryptococcosis, are additional diagnostic considerations.

When patients with AIDS and a past medical history of treated tuberculosis in the distant past present with a new pulmonary disorder, clinicians may be tempted to discount the diagnostic possibility of tuberculosis, especially when a chest radiograph is normal within a 2-year period. Tuberculosis, however, remains a distinctly likely explanation for illness in this clinical setting. Understanding how patients may acquire a "second episode" of tuberculosis requires a discussion of the general outcome of modern-day chemotherapy and new observations made by genetic "fingerprinting analysis."

Current treatment regimens for drug-sensitive tuberculosis have proved extremely effective in achieving initial bacterial sterilization of sputum. The relapse rate with these treatment protocols is reported to be less than 3.5% in nearly all clinical series, which has allowed modern-day, antituberculous regimens to be dubbed as "100% effective" therapy. Furthermore, multiple studies have demonstrated that when relapses (or "treatment failures") do occur, patients present with clinical evidence of pulmonary tuberculosis within 2 years after completion of therapy.

Considering the effectiveness of antituberculous chemotherapy, one might conclude that patients who develop another episode of tuberculosis later than 2 years after completion of therapy might be reinfected with the disease. In theory, however, reinfection with *M. tuberculosis* in a patient with a history of successfully treated tuberculosis has seemed to be extremely rare considering the immunity that would most likely develop during the initial infection. Indeed, William Stead, one of the pioneers of our modern understanding of tuberculosis, demonstrated in a landmark paper published nearly three decades ago that clinical disease was much more likely to result from endogenous reactivation than exogenous reinfection. Recent applications of molecular biology to patients with AIDS and tuberculosis, however, have allowed scientists to reexamine this issue in a new way.

Three recent studies provide evidence that challenges the prevailing notions about the development of clinical tuberculosis. One group, using restriction fragment length polymorphism (RFLP, or "DNA fingerprinting") analysis, demonstrated in patients with AIDS that what appeared to be tuberculosis relapses actually represented reinfection with different strains of *M. tuberculosis*. These strains were identified by the detection of distinct RFLP patterns from isolates collected during the initial and late infections. The importance of these observations relates to the high precision of RFLP analysis for determining uniqueness of *M. tuberculosis* isolates compared to older techniques that compared sensitivity patterns or phage types. RFLP patterns change much more slowly than sensitivity patterns or phage type characteristics and serve as reliable evidence of the importance of reinfection in patients who may appear to have tuberculosis due to reactivation or relapse.

Two other recent studies provide further evidence for the importance of reinfection. Data from San Francisco and New York indicate that as many as 40% of isolates within certain areas of these cities share the same RFLP fingerprint patterns. This observation further supports the concept that a great deal of disease is due to recent transmission and infection rather than relapse or reactivation. These data are beginning to make major contributions to our understanding of how tuberculosis is spread through populations. At present, however, much remains to be learned, and it is uncertain whether these observations can be applied to patients who do not have AIDS.

The present patient had a chest radiograph compatible with the diagnosis of tuberculosis and positive sputum smears for acid-fast bacilli. Cultures grew *M. tuberculosis* sensitive to all first-line drugs. In the absence of RFLP analysis on the current organism and the organism isolated from her tuberculosis episode 6 years earlier, it is impossible to know definitively whether her current tuberculosis was due to reactivation or reinfection. One might suspect, however, that the long interval between the two episodes indicates that reinfection occurred. She was placed on medications according to the ATS guidelines, with a good clinical response.

Clinical Pearls

1. When patients with AIDS and previously treated tuberculosis present with a new respiratory disorder, pulmonary tuberculosis is a likely diagnosis.

2. As many as 40% of cases of tuberculosis in patients with AIDS may be due to exogenous infection rather than reactivation of latent disease.

3. Prevailing notions about the development and spread of tuberculosis may change as RFLP analysis is extended. Our increasing awareness of the reinfection form of the disease places even greater emphasis on proper treatment and infection control.

REFERENCES

1. Stead WW. Pathogenesis of a first episode of chronic tuberculosis in man: recrudescence of residua of the primary infection or exogenous reinfection? Am Rev Respir Dis 1967:95:729–745.
2. Small PM, Shafer RW, Hopewell PC, et al. Exogenous reinfection with multidrug-resistant *Mycobacterium tuberculosis* in patients with advanced HIV infection. N Engl J Med 1993;328:1137–1144.
3. Small PM, Hopewell PC, Singh S, et al. The epidemiology of tuberculosis in San Francisco. A population-based study using conventional and molecular methods. N Engl J Med 1994;330:1703–1709.
4. Alland D, Kalkut GE, Moss A, et al. Transmission of tuberculosis in New York City. An analysis by DNA fingerprinting and conventional epidemiologic methods. N Engl J Med 1994;330:1710–1716.

PATIENT 71

A 33-year-old man with tuberculosis and noncompliance with therapy

A 33-year-old man was admitted after being issued an order for detention by the commissioner of health. He had a history of tuberculosis for the previous 3 years, during which time he had been sporadically compliant with therapy. For the last 2 years, he had been prescribed a regimen of cycloserine, ethionamide, ciprofloxacin, and kanamycin, but he admitted taking these medications rarely.

Physical Examination: Temperature 99.6°F, remainder of vital signs normal. General: thin man in no distress. Head: normal. Chest: rhonchi at the right apex. Heart: normal. Abdomen: normal. Extremities: normal. Neurologic: normal.

Laboratory Findings: CBC, serum electrolytes, liver function tests: normal. Chest radiograph: right upper lobe cavitary infiltrate. Sputum smear: negative for acid-fast bacilli. Sputum culture (sample obtained three months earlier): positive for *M. tuberculosis,* resistant to isoniazid, rifampin, ethambutol, streptomycin, and capreomycin.

Questions: What are the public health hazards posed by this patient? How should they be managed?

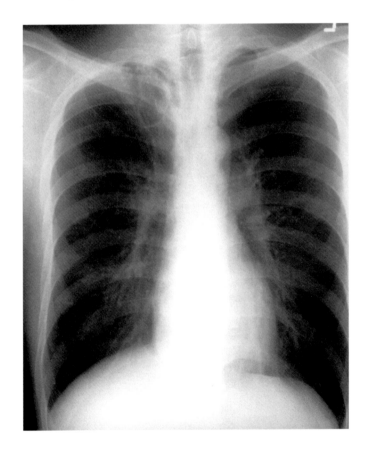

Diagnosis: Multidrug-resistant tuberculosis in a patient with demonstrated noncompliance with therapy.

Discussion: The problem of patient noncompliance with therapy for tuberculosis has existed since the first days of antituberculous chemotherapy, when patients were treated with painful daily injections (streptomycin) combined with up to 24 pills per day of a nauseating drug (para-aminosalicylic acid) for at least 18 months. Although most patients today are treated with more easily tolerated medications, treatment still consists of burdensome regimens of multiple drugs that need to be taken for a minimum of 6 months. Furthermore, effective treatment usually leads to resolution of symptoms within the first few weeks. Asymptomatic patients are thereafter tempted to discontinue their medications, which may not appear to be necessary from the patient's vantage point, for the duration of the recommended course of therapy.

In most clinical situations, the principle of patient autonomy allows competent patients to refuse medical treatment even if that refusal may result in the patient's death. In the management of patients with tuberculosis, however, noncompliance with antituberculous therapy raises special public health issues, due in part to the chronic nature of a disease in which the patient may remain infectious for months to years. Noncompliance not only may lead to an infectious relapse in a partially treated patient, but also may promote the emergence of infectious, multidrug-resistant tuberculosis that may respond to treatment in as few as 60% of patients. These outcomes result in a public health hazard. Consequently, many states have legislated limitations to the rights of patients with contagious tuberculosis to refuse medical therapy and thereby infect others. These laws must achieve their goal without unfairly impinging on the civil liberties of the noncompliant patient, while striking a balance between public health interests (the right not to be infected if infection can be avoided) and the rights of the individual patient to accept or refuse treatment. Most often, these efforts result in legislation that imposes enforced isolation, directly observed therapy (DOT) with antituberculous agents, or both.

A consensus exists, however, that a patient should not be punished for noncompliance due to certain circumstances beyond his or her control, such as lack of access to health care or inability to pay for medications. Therefore, most states have provisions for free medications, and many further provide "enablers" such as car fare to and from health care facilities, and, in some cases, even incentives such as meals or cash payments. DOT programs that provide supervised administration of medications in a clinic setting have been advocated as the standard of care by several authorities. Most programs currently in operation additionally have "outreach" workers who, when necessary, travel to the patient's residence, workplace, or, in extreme cases, to bars, "shooting galleries" or "crack houses" in order to administer medications.

Nonetheless, a small percentage of patients will not cooperate with these more aggressive attempts at promoting proper treatment. The recognition that these patients pose a significant public menace has led 42 states to initiate legislation that permits the commitment of recalcitrant tuberculosis patients to health care facilities. The Centers for Disease Control and Prevention (CDC) recently surveyed the tuberculosis control laws throughout the United States and made recommendations to address discrepancies between existing laws and previous guidelines for the control of tuberculosis. These recommendations emphasize that committing patients to inpatient treatment is a last resort in the attempt to treat noncompliant patients. A stepwise increase in the level of intervention should first be attempted, starting with DOT. This may be followed by DOT with enablers or incentives, then court-ordered DOT, before the determination is made that commitment should be sought for a noncompliant individual. Provisions should be made for certain circumstances of special urgency, such as enforced examination of patients suspected of having infectious tuberculosis, or emergency isolation and detention of patients known to have infectious disease. The duration of detention in many states is only until the patient becomes noninfectious; the recommendation of the CDC is that patients be detained until completely treated or until compliance with the remainder of the treatment regimen is assured. To ensure that the rights of the patient are maintained, any detention order to examine, isolate, or treat patients must meet due process requirements, and patients should have the right to legal counsel and to appeal decisions of detention.

Regarding the current patient, details of multiple instances of noncompliance with treatment, including mandated DOT, were submitted to the department of health. A detention order was obtained, and the patient was served with the order. He currently is being treated with the previous regimen, and his fever has resolved, cough has improved, and sputum smear positivity has decreased. When he is considered noninfectious, he will be transferred to a long-term health care facility specially designed for detained tuberculosis patients, where he will remain to complete a course of treatment.

Clinical Pearls

1. The right of an individual patient with tuberculosis to refuse treatment must be balanced against the right of the general public not to be infected by that individual.

2. The consequences of noncompliance with tuberculosis treatment, specifically the continuation of an infectious state and the potential for the development of a drug-resistant organism, impact on the patient's right to refuse treatment or isolation.

3. Most states have legislation that permits the involuntary commitment of tuberculous patients who refuse to comply with isolation procedures, treatment, or both; the same laws protect the patient by ensuring due process, legal counsel, and the right to appeal.

4. Involuntary commitment of noncompliant patients should be a last resort, after attempts at DOT in a clinic or by outreach workers have failed; circumstances beyond the patient's control (e.g. homelessness, serious illness) should be addressed first by the state, if they are the primary cause of noncompliance.

REFERENCES

1. Annas GJ. Control of tuberculosis—the law and the public's health. N Engl J Med 1993;328:585–588.
2. Iseman MD, Cohn DL, Sbarbaro JA. Directly observed treatment of tuberculosis. N Engl J Med 1993;328:576–578.
3. Willis BM, Schwartz LP, Knowlton SB. Tuberculosis control laws–United States, 1993. MMWR 1993;42:1–28.
4. New York City Health Code section 11.47.

PATIENT 72

A 47-year-old man with fever and abdominal swelling

A 47-year-old man was referred for evaluation of fever and a generalized, nonspecific abdominal pain of 3 weeks' duration. He also noted an increase in his abdominal girth. There was no history of alcohol use, viral hepatitis, or tuberculosis. He had moved from Panama 6 years earlier, and shared an apartment with several other immigrants.

Physical Examination: Temperature 100.4°F, remainder of vital signs normal. Head: normal. Chest: normal. Heart: normal. Abdomen: distended, positive fluid wave, no rebound, no discrete masses. Extremities: normal. Neurologic: normal.

Laboratory Findings: Hct 27.5%, WBC 6,900/μl, platelets 66,000/μl. Serum Na⁺ 130 mEq/L, K⁺ 3.4 mEq/L, Cl⁻ 99 mEq/L, HCO₃⁻ 22 mEq/L. Liver function tests: normal. Chest radiograph: normal. Tuberculin skin test: reactive to 12-mm induration. Abdominal paracentesis: serosanguinous fluid, RBC 10,560/μl, WBC 25/μl (76% lymphocytes, 19% neutrophils); glucose 104 mg/dl, total protein 4.0 g/dl. Gram stain: negative; acid-fast smear: negative.

Questions: What is the probable diagnosis? What therapy should be instituted?

Diagnosis: Tuberculous peritonitis.

Discussion: Although most patient series from the last several decades indicate that peritoneal tuberculosis is an unusual entity in the United States, recent reports suggest that this form of the disease is increasing in incidence in patients with HIV infection. It is uncertain, however, whether these patients have a particular risk for peritoneal tuberculosis or if this increased incidence is a consequence of the greater risk of extrapulmonary tuberculosis in general that is noted in patients with AIDS. In developing countries, peritoneal tuberculosis remains an important cause of ascites and the most common form of intra-abdominal tuberculosis.

Most patients develop peritoneal tuberculosis subsequent to local reactivation of an intra-abdominal focus of infection implanted during the primary hematogenous phase of the disease. Consequently, only 15% of patients with peritoneal tuberculosis have concomitant active pulmonary disease. Rarely, contiguous spread of infection from gastrointestinal or genitourinary organs is implicated in the pathogenesis of peritoneal tuberculosis.

Almost all patients with peritoneal tuberculosis present with abdominal swelling and discomfort. Although fever and weight loss are frequent complaints, systemic symptoms occur most often in patients who also have pulmonary involvement. Almost all patients have ascites at the time of presentation; only about 3% present with the "doughy" abdomen found in the dry, fibroadhesive form of peritoneal tuberculosis. About three-quarters of patients demonstrate a positive tuberculin reaction, while about one-half will have an abnormal chest radiograph, most of which represent inactive disease. Analysis of the peritoneal fluid reveals an exudate, usually with a white blood cell count of up to 4,000/µl, the majority of which are lymphocytes. The unusual finding of a neutrophil predominance in the ascitic fluid may be seen when peritoneal tuberculosis occurs in a patient receiving peritoneal dialysis. Additionally, patients with alcoholic cirrhosis, which causes a low protein ascites, and peritoneal tuberculosis may have peritoneal fluid proteins measured in the transudative range.

Ultrasound and CT examination of the abdomen can provide nonspecific but supportive diagnostic evidence of peritoneal tuberculosis. The CT finding of intra-abdominal adenopathy with low-density centers, usually in the mesenteric and peripancreatic areas, is particularly suggestive of intra-abdominal tuberculosis. CT appearance of ascites is usually that of a high-density, complex fluid collection, which may be loculated. Mesenteric and omental soft-tissue thickening is frequently observed.

Rapid diagnosis of peritoneal tuberculosis may be problematic, because as few as 3% of patients will have acid-fast organisms found on smear of ascitic fluid. Approximately 20% of cultures of ascitic fluid will be positive, although culture yields up to 80% have been reported when cultures are performed on the pellet of large volumes (> 1 L) of centrifuged ascitic fluid. Several articles have reported the utility of measuring adenosine deaminase activity in ascitic fluid, but reliability in the clinical application of this test remains unproven. Although blind percutaneous needle biopsy is a safe technique with yields above 50%, the diagnosis is usually made in this country by laparoscopy with direct peritoneal biopsy. This technique has a low complication rate and provides a very high diagnostic yield. In one series, 142 of 145 patients had a typical appearance of "miliary" tubercles studding the peritoneum or omentum, and granulomas were found on 100% of biopsies, whereas acid-fast bacilli were demonstrated in 74%.

Medical treatment for peritoneal tuberculosis is no different from treatment for pulmonary disease, and equivalent success rates should be anticipated.

The present patient was started on a standard four-drug regimen for tuberculosis after he refused any further work-up. Cultures of the ascitic fluid subsequently grew *M. tuberculosis*. The patient was lost to follow-up after 3 months of therapy.

Clinical Pearls

1. Peritoneal tuberculosis is uncommon in industrialized nations but remains a significant cause of ascites in developing countries.

2. While most patients with peritoneal tuberculosis have lymphocytic-predominant exudative ascites, atypical fluid findings include a neutrophilic predominance in association with peritoneal dialysis and low protein ascites in the presence of cirrhosis.

3. CT findings suggestive of peritoneal tuberculosis include high-density, complex-appearing ascites accompanied by enlarged, low-density intra-abdominal lymph nodes.

4. The laparoscopic appearance of peritoneal studding with miliary tubercles is suggestive of peritoneal tuberculosis, and biopsy of the lesions is usually confirmatory.

REFERENCES

1. Hulnick DH, Megibow AJ, Naidich DP, et al. Abdominal tuberculosis: CT evaluation. Radiology 1985;157:199–204.
2. Manohar A, Simjee AE, Haffejee AA, Pettengell KE. Symptoms and investigative findings in 145 patients with tuberculous peritonitis diagnosed by peritoneoscopy and biopsy over a five year period. Gut 1990;31:1130–1132.
3. Rosengart TK, Coppa GF. Abdominal mycobacterial infections in immunocomprised patients. Am J Surg 1990;159:125–131.
4. Bhargava DK, Shriniwas, Chopra P, et al. Peritoneal tuberculosis: laparoscopic patterns and its diagnostic accuracy. Am J Gastroenterol 1992;87:109–112.
5. Marshall JB. Tuberculosis of the gastrointestinal tract and peritoneum. Am J Gastroenterol 1993;88:989–999.

PATIENT 73

A 42-year-old man with the onset of psychosis during treatment for multidrug-resistant tuberculosis

A 42-year-old homeless man with a history of alcoholism and multidrug-resistant tuberculosis was transferred from another hospital for evaluation of paranoid ideation. He had a 4-year history of tuberculosis and poor compliance with drug therapy. Six weeks before transfer, he had been admitted elsewhere for management of fevers, night sweats, cough productive of green sputum, and weight loss. Sputum smears were positive for acid-fast bacilli and therapy was initiated with ethambutol, streptomycin, ciprofloxacin, and ethionamide. A sputum culture from an evaluation 2 months earlier became available and indicated that the patient had a strain of *M. tuberculosis* that was resistant to all first-line antituberculous drugs. Ethambutol and streptomycin were stopped, and cycloserine, pyridoxine, para-aminosalicylic acid, and capreomycin were added to ciprofloxacin and ethionamide. The patient's cough slowly improved but he gradually became withdrawn and paranoid, stopping almost all verbal interaction with staff members. He then began experiencing auditory hallucinations.

Physical Examination: Afebrile. General: minimally cooperative, disheveled, poor eye contact. Chest: decreased breath sounds and bronchophony throughout left lung field. Abdomen: nontender, no hepatosplenomegaly. Neurologic: oriented to person only; cranial nerve, motor and sensory exams intact and nonfocal, no meningismus.

Laboratory Findings: Hct 32%, WBC 4,200/μl. Electrolytes and renal indices: normal. Aspartate aminotransferase 67 IU/L, alanine aminotransferase 92 IU/L. Sputum: positive for acid-fast bacilli. HIV test: negative. Chest radiograph: shown below. Head CT: mild cortical atrophy. Lumbar puncture: acellular, protein 35 mg/dl, glucose 65 mg/dl, Gram stains and acid-fast stains negative.

Question: What is the cause of this patient's change in mental status?

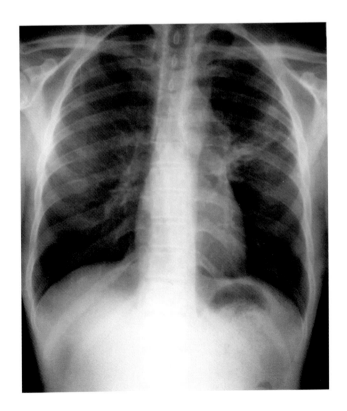

Diagnosis: Cycloserine-induced psychosis.

Discussion: Antituberculous agents such as cycloserine, ethionamide, and para-aminosalicylic acid have received the designation of "second-line drugs" because they tend to be both less effective in treating tuberculosis and more toxic than first-line agents. The use of second-line agents becomes necessary in pulmonary tuberculosis when patients develop disease with multi-drug resistant strains. In such instances, familiarity with the toxicities of these drugs is essential in order to minimize the incidence and severity of side effects and to maximize patient compliance.

Cycloserine is a bacteriostatic drug used at a dose of 15 mg/kg, with a maximum dose of 1 g/day. Its most significant and most common side effects involve the central nervous system, and are related to the drug's ability to easily cross the meninges. Neurologic reactions range from relatively mild clinical manifestations, such as insomnia, inability to concentrate, headache, and short-term memory difficulties, to severe adverse reactions, such as seizures, profound personality changes, and overt psychosis. Severe depression is of particular concern, and requires careful monitoring, because suicides have occurred in patients treated with this agent. Patients with a prior history of psychiatric problems are at increased risk for suffering the psychological complications of cycloserine. Peripheral neuropathies can also occur in patients treated with cycloserine, especially when it is used in combination with isoniazid.

Because cycloserine is renally excreted, the risk for adverse drug reactions increases in the setting of renal insufficiency. Patients with impaired renal function should undergo monitoring of plasma drug levels. Maintaining cycloserine concentrations below 30 μg/ml reduces the incidence of toxicity. Pyridoxine may decrease the risk for seizures and peripheral neuropathy, and should be given at a dose of 50 mg for every 250 mg of cycloserine.

Ethionamide is related to isoniazid, both being a derivative of isonicotinic acid. It is quite active against *M. tuberculosis* in vitro, but its usefulness is greatly restrained by side effects, particularly the gastrointestinal disorders experienced by a majority of patients. Nausea, vomiting, anorexia, abdominal pain, belching, flatulence, and metallic taste frequently render the medication intolerable. The usual dose is 15 mg/kg, with a maximum dose of 1 g/day. If therapy is initiated with the full dose, gastrointestinal symptoms are often so severe that patients will refuse to take ethionamide again. The wiser strategy is to start with one 250-mg pill per day, and increase the daily dose by one pill every 5–7 days. The daily dose may be divided, and administering the drug at bedtime with an antiemetic or hypnotic may enhance tolerance.

Neurologic side effects are additional common adverse reactions to ethionamide. Patients may experience headache, restlessness, dizziness, depression, and seizures. Hepatoxicity occurs in about 5% of patients, so monthly monitoring of transaminases is recommended. Arthralgias, impotence, irregular menses, and hair loss can also occur. Hypothyroidism, which occurs more frequently when ethionamide is used in combination with para-aminosalicylic acid, is an important side effect to keep in mind.

Para-aminosalicylic acid is a bacteriostatic agent that must be used in high doses to be clinically effective. The standard dose is 150 mg/kg, with a maximum daily dose of 12 g. Standard regimens translate to as many as 24 large tablets per day, which is a daunting prospect in itself for most patients. The most common side effects are nausea, vomiting, and diarrhea. These gastrointestinal symptoms make the combination of para-aminosalicylic acid and ethionamide particularly noxious for most patients. Para-aminosalicylic acid is now available in a granular form that may be more easily tolerated. Remember in treating patients with congestive heart failure that para-aminosalicylic acid contains a considerable sodium load. Hypersensitivity reactions occur in up to 10% of patients, and hepatotoxicity may rarely occur.

The present patient was considered to be experiencing a neuropsychiatric reaction to cycloserine, which was discontinued on admission. The patient returned to his baseline mental status within 5 days.

Clinical Pearls

1. Cycloserine can cause serious psychiatric disturbances, sometimes severe enough to lead to suicide, especially in patients with a previous history of such disorders.

2. Pyridoxine should be given at a dose of 50 mg per 250 mg of cycloserine to help prevent seizures and peripheral neuropathy.

3. To improve gastrointestinal tolerance of ethionamide, the dose should be gradually increased from one pill per day; administration with an antiemetic or hypnotic at bedtime may also be helpful.

4. Hypothyroidism may be caused by either ethionamide or para-aminosalicylic acid, and the incidence is increased when both drugs are contained in the same regimen.

5. Administration of the granular form of para-aminosalicylic acid may decrease the adverse gastrointestinal effects.

REFERENCES

1. Pattyn SR, Janssens L, Bourlan J, et al. Hepatotoxicity of the combination of rifampin-ethionamide in the treatment of multibacillary leprosy. Int J Lepr Other Mycobact Dis 1984;52:1–6.
2. Holdiness MR. Adverse cutaneous reactions to antituberculous drugs. Int J Dermatol 1985 24:280–285.
3. Iseman MD, Madsen LA. Drug-resistant tuberculosis. Clin Chest Med 1989;10:341–353.
4. Yew WW, Wong CF, Wong PC, et al. Adverse neurological reactions in patients with multidrug-resistant pulmonary tuberculosis after coadministration of cycloserine and ofloxacin. Clin Infect Dis 1994;17:288–289.
2. Aranda CP. Second-line agents: para-aminosalicylic acid, ethionamide, cycloserine, and thioacetazone. In: Rom WN, Garay SM, eds. Tuberculosis. Boston: Little, Brown, 1995.

PATIENT 74

A 25-year-old man with an abnormal chest radiograph and a rectal fistula

A 25-year-old Asian male was referred for evaluation of a positive tuberculin skin test and an abnormal chest radiograph. He had been evaluated 1 week earlier for a perineal fistula and scheduled for biopsy and fistulotomy. An abnormal preoperative chest radiograph, however, prompted cancellation of surgery and placement of the tuberculin test. He denied cough, fever, night sweats, or weight loss. There was no history of a previous tuberculin test or close contact with an active case of tuberculosis.

Physical Examination: Vital signs: normal. General: comfortable. Chest: clear to auscultation and percussion. Heart: normal. Abdomen: no organomegaly. Rectal: draining fistula with purulent exudate.

Laboratory Findings: CBC, serum electrolytes, liver function tests: normal. Chest radiograph: fibrotic infiltrate in the right upper lobe. Sputum AFB smear: negative.

Clinical Course: The patient was started on multidrug chemotherapy because of the abnormal chest radiograph that was suggestive of tuberculosis and the positive tuberculin test result. The perineal fistula was considered to be an unrelated problem. All sputum cultures were subsequently found to be negative for *M. tuberculosis*. Five weeks later, the patient returned to his surgeon, who noted that the perineal fistula had closed spontaneously. The patient completed a total of four months of multidrug therapy in accordance with ATS recommendations for treatment of patients with radiograph evidence of old untreated tuberculosis and negative sputum cultures. Two months after discontinuation of drug therapy, the patient noted a recurrence of the rectal fistula. A culture of the fistula drainage was performed and found to be positive for *M. tuberculosis*.

Questions: What should be the management of the patient's rectal fistula? What errors in therapy occurred?

Diagnosis: Tuberculous rectal fistula (fistula-in-ano).

Discussion: Tuberculosis of the gastrointestinal tract is a relatively uncommon manifestation of extrapulmonary disease in the chemotherapy era. Although peritoneal tuberculosis accounts for 3.8% of extrapulmonary cases of tuberculosis, tuberculous involvement of the gut itself occurs even less frequently. When gastrointestinal disease does develop, it usually affects younger age groups, although a second but somewhat smaller incidence peak occurs in old age.

Gastrointestinal tuberculosis is a form of reactivation disease that arises in foci of infection that developed during the initial or "primary" stage of the disease. Other mechanisms of gastrointestinal infection, however, may also exist. Acid-fast organisms may be coughed up in sputum from pulmonary sites of infection and swallowed, thereby innoculating the gastrointestinal tract. This mechanism may account for the fact that active pulmonary tuberculosis is a common finding in patients with gastrointestinal sites of the disease.

The terminal ileum is by far the most common site for gastrointestinal tuberculosis. Tuberculosis of the rectum has long been recognized as a distinct clinical entity, although its incidence has always been uncommon even in the pre-chemotherapeutic era. Tuberculosis of the rectum is uncommon and, when it occurs, usually is found in a patient with pulmonary tuberculosis. Considered the other way, however, mycobacterial infection accounted for up to 80% of the etiologies of rectal fistulae in the pre-chemotherapeutic era.

Currently, tuberculous fistula-in-ano still accounts for a small but clinically important percentage of rectal fistulae, particularly in underdeveloped countries where tuberculosis is hyperendemic. One series of 122 patients with fistulae-in-ano undergoing surgery during a 5-year period included 19 patients (15.6%) with rectal tuberculosis. A second series of 82 cases found 4 (5%) patients with perineal fistulae caused by tuberculosis. Two distinct types of tuberculosis anal fistula have been reported in the older literature: a verrucous growth extending from the perianal region into the anal canal, and the more common ulcerative type with sharp edges and a mucopurulent discharge. The patient presented here fits the latter type.

The diagnosis of a tuberculous rectal fistula requires the demonstration of granulomas in the fistula tract or positive cultures for *M. tuberculosis* from the fistula drainage. The differential diagnosis include granulomatous colitis and Crohn's disease. Of these diagnoses, Crohn's disease involving the rectum and tuberculosis can have extremely similar clinical presentations. Both disorders may involve any segment of the gastrointestinal tract, produce "skip" lesions, and present with pain. Indeed, the similarities between these two conditions have caused early investigators to ascribe the etiology of Crohn's disease to atypical manifestations of mycobacterial infection. The treatment of tuberculosis rectal fistula is medical, with the initiation of a 9–12-month course of antituberculous drug therapy, although some patients may require excision of the fistula if they fail to respond.

Although the present patient had classic manifestations of a tuberculous rectal fistula, the clinicians failed to make an association between the abnormal chest radiograph, positive tuberculin test, and perineal disease. Interestingly, despite responding to the initial 4-month course of chemotherapy, the rectal fistula failed to improve upon reinitiation of antituberculous drug therapy. He underwent surgical excision, and pathologic specimens demonstrated granulomas and positive growth for *M. tuberculosis* sensitive to all available drugs.

Clinical Pearls

1. Tuberculous rectal fistulae should be a leading differential diagnostic consideration in patients at high risk for active tuberculosis who present with perineal lesions.
2. Patients presenting with the clinical manifestations of Crohn's disease should be evaluated for gastrointestinal tuberculosis if a chest radiograph is suggestive of active or healed tuberculous disease.
3. Tuberculous rectal fistulae will usually respond to medical therapy, but if purulent drainage persists several months into therapy, surgical excision may be required.

REFERENCES

1. Ani AN, Solanke TF. Anal fistula: a review of 82 cases. Dis Colon Rectum 1976;19:51–55.
2. Shukla HS, Gupta SC, Singh G, Singh PA. Tubercular fistula in ano. Br J Surg 1988;75:38–9.
3. Healy JC, Gorman S, Kumar PJ. Case report: tuberculous colitis mimicking Crohn's disease. Clin Radiol 1992;46:131–132.
4. Lavy A, Militianu D, Eidelman S. Diseases of the intestine mimicking Crohn's disease. J Clin Gastro 1992;15:17–23.
5. Harland RW, Varkey B. Anal tuberculosis: report of two cases and a review of the literature. Am J Gastroenterol 1992; 87:1488–1491.

PATIENT 75

A 3-month-old boy whose father has active pulmonary tuberculosis

A 3-month-old boy was brought to the pediatric clinic by his parents to assess his risk for tuberculosis. The infant's father had been diagnosed 2 weeks earlier with active pulmonary tuberculosis, and placed on therapy with isoniazid, rifampin, pyrazinamide, and ethambutol. The father's most recent sputum examination was negative for acid-fast bacilli. The child had been healthy and met growth and development milestones for age. The mother had a positive tuberculin skin test but was asymptomatic with a normal chest radiograph.

Physical Examination: Vital signs: normal. General: healthy-appearing male infant. The remainder of the physical examination was normal.

Laboratory Findings: CBC and liver function tests: normal. Chest radiograph: normal.

Questions: How should the infant be evaluated? What therapy, if any, should be given?

Diagnosis: Household tuberculosis exposure of an infant.

Discussion: Contact tracing is an important element of any tuberculosis control program and an effective way to limit the spread of the disease. The chance of developing tuberculosis is high among close contacts of active cases, and thus all close contacts (particularly household contacts) should be sought out and evaluated for both infection and active disease. Adults who contact active, smear-positive tuberculosis cases should be evaluated with a tuberculin skin test and a directed history aimed at eliciting symptoms of active disease. Asymptomatic adult contacts who have a tuberculin skin test with less than 5 mm of induration do not require preventive therapy. The contact should be followed closely, however, and the tuberculin test repeated three months later. If the repeat skin test is positive, the contact should be placed on isoniazid preventive therapy if no evidence of active disease exists.

Adult contacts with an initially positive tuberculin skin test should have a chest radiograph obtained. Those with normal radiographs will usually be candidates for isoniazid preventive therapy, regardless of age. Those with abnormal chest radiographs should be evaluated for active disease.

Contact investigations involving HIV-infected persons, other immunocompromised persons, and children represent special situations. HIV-infected contacts of active cases of tuberculosis should undergo tuberculin skin testing. If induration is less than 5 mm and a simultaneous anergy panel is reactive, many experts recommend instituting isoniazid preventive therapy for at least 3 months after the contact has ended, at which time the skin test should be repeated. If the test still shows less than 5 mm of induration, isoniazid may be stopped. If the skin test is positive at any time (more than 5 mm of induration), isoniazid prophylaxis should be administered for a total duration of 12 months. A negative tuberculin test in the presence of anergy requires special considerations in patients with HIV infection.

Children under 5 years of age who are contacts of a smear-positive case of tuberculosis should be treated with isoniazid preventive therapy at a dose of 10 mg/kg, regardless of the result of the tuberculin skin test. This recommendation exists because 2–10 weeks may be required for the tuberculin skin test to become positive, and small children are extremely vulnerable to rapid progression of active tuberculosis. In children started on isoniazid preventive therapy with initially negative skin tests, the test should be repeated 3 months after isoniazid was started. If the skin test is still negative, therapy can be discontinued, as long as the child is no longer in close contact with an infectious case of tuberculosis.

For children who are close contacts of active cases (particularly active drug-resistant cases) and who cannot be safely protected from exposure (the source case is not taking medication or remains smear positive despite therapy), vaccination with BCG may be considered. Considerable debate exists about the utility of this vaccine, which is considered to be moderately effective at best. It may be the only preventive measure available, however, in such clinical settings. If a child is BCG vaccinated, a tuberculin skin test should be done 8 weeks afterward, and if there is less than 5 mm of induration, vaccination should be repeated.

In the past, the tine (multiple puncture) test was widely used as a tool to evaluate tuberculosis infection in children. The Centers for Disease Control and Prevention, the American Thoracic Society, and the American Academy of Pediatrics, however, recommend that this test not be performed because of poor standardization of the application and interpretation of the multipuncture technique.

The present child had a negative tuberculin test and was started on isoniazid preventive therapy. The skin test was still negative 3 months later. Because the father complied with drug therapy and felt well, the child's isoniazid was discontinued.

Clinical Pearls

1. Household contacts of patients with active tuberculosis should be thoroughly evaluated for preventive therapy because of their high risk of contracting the disease.

2. Certain extremely vulnerable persons who are contacts of an active case initially should be given isoniazid preventive therapy regardless of the initial tuberculin skin test result. Such patients include persons with HIV infection and very young children.

3. BCG vaccination may be indicated as preventive therapy if the source case remains infectious and a child contact cannot be adequately protected from the infectious risk.

REFERENCES

1. Nolan RJ. Childhood tuberculosis in North Carolina: a study of the opportunities for intervention in the transmission of tuberculosis to children. Am J Pub Health 1986;76:26–30.
2. Nemir RL, O'Hare D. Tuberculosis in children 10 years of age and younger: three decades of experience during the chemotherapeutic era. Pediatrics 1991;88:236–241.
3. Starke JR, Jacobs RF, Jereb J. Resurgence of tuberculosis in children. J Pediatr 1992;120:839–855.
4. Vallejo JG, Ong LT, Starke JR. Clinical features, diagnosis, and treatment of tuberculosis in children. Pediatrics 1994;94:1–7.
5. American Academy of Pediatrics/Committee on Infectious Diseases. Screening for tuberculosis in infants and children. Pediatrics 1994;93:131–134.

INDEX

Page numbers in **boldface** indicate complete cases.